Essentials of Neurological and Neurosurgical Nursing

Essentials of Neurological and Neurosurgical Nursing

Second Edition

TP Prema MS (N) DPN PhD
Visiting Professor in Psychiatric Nursing
New Jersey, USA

KF Graicy RN RM BSc (N) MSc (N)
Professor, Shyamala Reddy College of Nursing
Bengaluru, Karnataka, India

Foreword
G Kasthuri

JAYPEE

JAYPEE BROTHERS MEDICAL PUBLISHERS
The Health Sciences Publisher
New Delhi | London

JAYPEE **Jaypee Brothers Medical Publishers (P) Ltd**

Headquarters
EMCA House
23/23-B, Ansari Road, Daryaganj
New Delhi 110 002, India
Landline: +91-11-23272143, +91-11-23272703
+91-11-23282021, +91-11-23245672
E-mail: jaypee@jaypeebrothers.com

Corporate Office
4838/24, Ansari Road, Daryaganj
New Delhi 110 002, India
Phone: +91-11-43574357
Fax: +91-11-43574314
E-mail: jaypee@jaypeebrothers.com

Overseas Office
J.P. Medical Ltd
83 Victoria Street, London
SW1H 0HW (UK)
Phone: +44 20 3170 8910
E-mail: info@jpmedpub.com

EU GPSR Authorised Representative
Logos Europe, 9 rue Nicolas Poussin
17000, La Rochelle, France
Phone: +33 (0) 6 67 93 73 78
E-mail: contact@logoseurope.eu

Website: www.jaypeebrothers.com
Website: www.jaypeedigital.com

Inquiries for bulk sales may be solicited at: jaypee@jaypeebrothers.com

Essentials of Neurological and Neurosurgical Nursing

First Edition : 2002

Second Edition : **2013**

Reprint: **2026**

ISBN : 978-93-5025-935-1

Printed at: Samrat Offset Pvt. Ltd.

To

Our Parents and Nursing Society

Foreword

It is my pleasure to write the Foreword for the book *Essentials of Neurological and Neurosurgical Nursing* written by Dr (Mrs) TP Prema and Mrs KF Graicy. Perhaps, it may be the first venture of its kind from Indian authors.

This book is the result of keen interest of authors in improving the nursing care of patient with neurological problems.

This book deals with most common as well as rarely found neuro conditions.

This book has been organized into several small units which discuss the definition, etiology, pathology, signs and symptoms, and management, especially the role of nurses in the management, based on the nursing process approach.

The language is simple and easy-to-understand, short and well-concised. This book is written in a point-to-point stepwise pattern, which will help the students to understand easily.

I am sure this book will not only be useful for the nursing students but will also serve as a handbook and a lifelong companion to the nursing professionals.

I am confident that the book will fulfill its aim of raising the standard of nursing care of patients with neurological and neurosurgical problems. I compliment the authors for their maiden venture and wish them every success.

G Kasthuri MSc (N) PhD
Principal
Government College of Nursing, Fort
Bengaluru, Karnataka, India

Preface to the Second Edition

It gives us immense pleasure and satisfaction to introduce the second edition of *Essentials of Neurological and Neurosurgical Nursing*. Many nursing students expressed the usefulness of this book as handy reference. We are happy to incorporate some of the corrections and suggestions which are received from nursing professionals.

This edition has one new chapter Nursing Management of Patient with Ventilator (Chapter 27). It has sharpened the focus on presenting most current, relevant, practical, concise information on neuronursing.

In fact, this book is the outcome of the felt need of the authors. Having worked in the National Institute of Mental Health and Neurosciences (NIMHANS) for the last three decades and a few years in Neurocenter of NIMHANS, we experienced the non-availability of books on Neuroscience Nursing especially by Indian authors. So, with lots of apprehension and equal amount of enthusiasm, we have taken up this project.

Neuroscience nursing has undergone many changes in the last few years, along with the changes happened in neurological and neurosurgical practices. The different authors books, written at different stages, are influencing neuroscience nursing also. In the last three decades, there are Neuroscience Nursing books written by nursing professionals but a few in number. We hope the availability of more number of books can strengthen the knowledge and practices of nurses in this field in future.

This text is arranged in four units, which includes 27 chapters. **Unit One** has five chapters, discussing the overview of neuronursing and its new challenges, review of anatomy and physiology of nervous system, neurological examination—nurses' role, diagnostic procedures in neurological conditions—nurses' role, and interventional neuroradiology—nurses' role. The objective of this unit is to make the nurses aware of the normal anatomy, the nurses' role in different investigations and examinations in neuroscience. This knowledge should, in turn, help the nurses to identify the alarming signs of different neurological conditions, which need immediate action.

Unit Two has three chapters. Major number of neurological conditions are due to the deficits occurring from various disease entities. So, this unit explains a few of such conditions and its nursing management. Mainly management of patients with unconsciousness, urinary incontinence and aphasia are discussed in this unit.

Unit Three has 14 chapters. It covers almost all neurological conditions with their definition, etiology, signs and symptoms, investigations and diagnostic procedures, management in general and nursing management in particular. It is also dealing with all neurosurgical conditions and its management.

Unit Four has five chapters. It talks about the common drugs used in neurosurgical conditions, nurses' role in rehabilitating the patients' neurological, neurosurgical conditions, summary of common problems identified by nurses in those conditions, nursing diagnosis and the nursing intervention. One chapter of this unit gives the role of nurse in the prevention of the neurological and neurosurgical conditions. The last chapter is a new chapter which gives the nursing management of patients who need ventilator care.

This book gives the nursing care of almost all conditions seen in neurocenters. Not only the books but also the experience in neurocenter of NIMHANS, the exposure to the Institute of Neurological Sciences Southern General Hospital, Glasgow (UK) and Western General Hospital, Edinburgh (UK), Queen's Medical Center, Hawaii (USA), Kapiolani Hospital, Hawaii (USA), helped the authors to complete this work.

The authors used simple language, in brief length to explain the essentials of neuronursing in this particular text. This can be used by the general nursing students, nurses working in neuro-centers, students undergoing diploma in neuronursing, diploma in psychiatric nursing, nurses sponsored by WHO (World Health Organization) and KSHDP (Karnataka State Health Development Program) who undergo short-term training programs in neuro-nursing. This book can be used even by the undergraduate students in nursing courses and any other personnel who wish to have short-term training program in neuronursing.

We acknowledge our sincere thanks to the ward supervisors and nurses of neurocenters for their contributions of the practical experience, which helped us to complete the work successfully. We also thank the Neurologists, Neurosurgeons, Radiologists and other professionals who were directly or indirectly responsible for the completion of the project.

We thank Prof M Gourie Devi, Director/Vice-Chancellor of NIMHANS (Deemed University), Bengaluru, Karnataka, India for her kind words of encouragement. We also thank Dr (Mrs) K Reddamma, Professor and HOD of Nursing, NIMHANS, Dr KVR Shastry, Professor of Neurosurgery, Dr P Kodandaram, Additional Professor of Clinical Psychology, Mr AV Ramaswamy (Assistant Administrative Officer), for their encouragement and support for writing this book.

We place our deepest gratitude towards Dr (Mrs) G Kasthuri, Principal, Government College of Nursing, Fort, Bengaluru, Karnataka, India for her good self for writing the Foreword for this book. In spite of her busy schedule and the short notice from our side, she extended her sincere encouragement and made herself to write a well-worded Foreword for this attempt.

Finally, we record our thanks to all our family members and well-wishers who were with us from the day one to the completion of this work with their constant and commendable encouragement.

We thank M/s Jaypee Brothers Medical Publishers (P) Ltd, for undertaking the publication of this book and fulfilling the requirement of all nursing students and nurses working with neuropatients.

We are sure that this book will be useful for the nursing community who work with patients of neurological and neurosurgical problems.

TP Prema
KF Graicy

Preface to the First Edition

This book is the outcome of the felt need of the authors. Having worked in the National Institute of Mental Health and Neurosciences (NIMHANS) for the last two decades and a few years in Neurocenter of NIMHANS, we experienced the non-availability of books on Neuroscience Nursing especially by Indian authors. So with lots of apprehension and equal amount of enthusiasm, we have taken up this project.

Neuroscience nursing has undergone many changes in the last few years, along with the changes happened in neurological and neurosurgical practices. The different authors books, written at different stages, are influencing neuroscience nursing also. In the last two decades, there are Neuroscience Nursing books written by nursing professionals but a few in number. We hope the availability of more number of books can strengthen the knowledge and practices of nurses in this field in future.

This text is arranged in 4 units, which includes 26 chapters. The 1st unit has 5 chapters, discussing the overview of neuronursing and its new challenges, review of anatomy and physiology of nervous system, neurological examination—nurses' role, diagnostic procedures in neurological conditions—nurses' role, and interventional neuroradiology—nurses' role. The objective of this unit is to make the nurses aware of the normal anatomy, the nurses' role in different investigations and examination in neuroscience. This knowledge should, in turn, help the nurses to identify the alarming signs of different neurological conditions, which need immediate action.

The 2nd unit has 3 chapters. Major number of neurological conditions are due to the deficits occurring from various disease entities. So this unit explains a few of such conditions and its nursing management. Mainly management of patients with unconsciousness, urinary incontinence and aphasia are discussed in this unit.

The 3rd unit has 14 chapters. It covers almost all neurological conditions with their definition, etiology, signs and symptoms, investigations and diagnostic procedures, management in general and nursing management in particular. It is also dealing with all neurosurgical conditions and its management.

The 4th unit has 4 chapters. It talks about the common drugs used in neurosurgical conditions, nurses' role in rehabilitating the patients' neurological, neurosurgical conditions, summary of common problems identified by nurses in those conditions, nursing diagnosis and the nursing intervention. The last chapter of this unit gives the role of nurse in the prevention of the neurological and neurosurgical conditions.

This book gives the nursing care of almost all conditions seen in neurocenter. Not only the books but also the experience in neurocenter of NIMHANS, the exposure to the Institute of Neurological Sciences Southern General Hospital, Glasgow (UK) and Western General Hospital, Edinburgh (UK), Queen's Medical Center, Hawaii (USA), Kapiolani Hospital, Hawaii (USA), helped the authors to complete this work.

The authors used simple language, in brief length to explain the essentials of neuronursing in this particular text. This can be used by the general nursing students, nurses working in neurocenters, students undergoing diploma in neuronursing, diploma in psychiatric nursing, nurses sponsored by WHO (World Health Organization) and KSHDP (Karnataka State Health Development Program) who undergo short-term training programs in neuronursing. This book can be used even by the undergraduate students in nursing courses and any other personnel who wish to have short-term training program in neuronursing.

We acknowledge our sincere thanks to the ward supervisors and nurses of neurocenter for their contributions from the practical experience, which helped us to complete the work successfully. We also thank the Neurologists, Neurosurgeons, Radiologists and other professionals who were directly or indirectly responsible for the completion of the project.

We thank Prof M Gourie Devi, Director/Vice-Chancellor of NIMHANS (Deemed University), Bengaluru, Karnataka, India for her kind words of encouragement. We also thank Dr HM Gangadharaiah, Professor and HOD of Nursing NIMHANS, Dr KVR Shastry, Professor of Neurosurgery, Dr P Kodandaram,

Additional Professor of Clinical Psychology, Mr AV Ramaswamy (Assistant Administrative Officer) for their encouragement and support for writing this book.

We place our deepest gratitude towards Dr (Mrs) G Kasthuri, Principal, Government College of Nursing, Fort, Bengaluru, Karnataka, India for her good self for writing the Foreword for this book. In spite of her busy schedule and the short notice from our side, she extended her sincere encouragement and made herself to write a well-worded Foreword for this attempt.

Finally, we record our thanks to all our family members and well-wishers who were with us from the day one to the completion of this work with their constant and commendable encouragement.

We thank M/s Jaypee Brothers Medical Publishers (P) Ltd, for undertaking the publication of this book and fulfilling the requirement of all nursing students and nurses working with neuropatients.

We are sure that this book will be useful for the nursing community who work with patients of neurological and neurosurgical problems.

TP Prema
KF Graicy

Contents

Unit One

Unit Two

Unit Three

Unit Four

1

Overview of Neuronursing and its New Challenges

Unit One

Nursing or caring the sick is as old as the world itself. Family members, servants, friends, neighbors and religious groups cared the ill individuals as and when required. Then few people took up the job of nursing for their livelihood. Florence Nightingale provided a light to these group of women, a different dimension of their work, and therefore Florence Nightingale is known as the mother of modern nursing. Nursing has taken many other shapes as it started having a written curriculum to follow, has a definite period for practical experience and also the need to appear for an examination, before a certificate is issued.

The present-day nursing is an encounter with a client and his or her family wherein the nurse observes, supports, communicates, administers and teaches. The nurse also has the duty of her own independent diagnosis, intervention and evaluation of what she carries out for patients. She is also involved in research to improve the nursing management by forming nursing theory.

Other changes happened in nursing are according to the changes occurred in the medical and surgical services. These two basic concepts branched out enormously to its minute dimension. Among these developments, one of the important event is the invasion of neurology from medical science and neurosurgery from surgical science. Faster developments happened in neuroscience and 1990s was called as the decade of brain.

If the literature of the neuronursing is reviewed for last hundred years, it can be divided into three periods, i.e. early, transitional, and modern. In the early period, the neuronursing textbooks were written by neurophysicians. Those books were based on medical and surgical nursing and the literature reflected the dependent nature of nursing. In the second period, namely the transitional period, physicians and nurses were co-authors reflecting a trend towards interdependency of nursing practice. In the third, i.e. the modern period the nurses became independent authors of books written on neurological and neurosurgical nursing.

If one reviews the practice of neuronursing started out from the merely carrying out the doctors' orders. In 1970, the textbook written by Brunner and Sudharths placed emphasis on the nurses' role in assessment of the neurological patients by nurses. This also stated the plan of care including the nursing management of unconscious patient with objectives, principles and rationale for care. Here the nursing intervention were directed by data obtained from assessment of the patient and family and less by intuition and physicians' direction.

In 1975, Smith and Germain wrote about the clinical management by nurses for the patients with increased intracranial pressure. It listed the actions which the nurses can take during the management of patients with increased intracranial pressure. They are:

- Check vital signs every 30 minutes.
- Check the level of consciousness and pupillary reaction.
- Check for paralysis.
- Give breathing by mouth.
- Elevate the head end of the bed 30° angle.
- Maintain patients' head to the side.

Later, the different editions of textbook written by Joanne V. Hickay included the individual chapters on different neurological conditions, e.g. chapter on increased intracranial pressure, chapter on unconscious patient, etc.

Problems Faced by Nurses

Though the texts are available about the responsibilities of nurses, nurses do not use these texts to practice independently. They go for the old routine of carrying out the physicians' orders. Nursing text whether it is written by physicians or nurses, do not generally mention about the nursing management. Exception to this style are worthy of mentioning. Roger Bannister's revision of Brain's Clinical Neurology (1978) contained a very small section on nursing management of unconscious patient. Another example is, literature written by James R Howe, titled "Patient Care in Neurosurgery".

Observations regarding nursing care were extensive and spread in the text rather than clustered in a small section at the end of the each chapter. So now enough literature is available for neuronurses to take care of patients with different neurological or neurosurgical conditions. In practice, the nurse has few changes in her side such as preparing and assisting in the procedures like CT scan, MRI and Interventional radiology. In her neurosurgical operation theater, the nurse has different new equipments which she has to get acquainted. Laser and gamma knife are two such equipments which are not available in many neurosurgical operation theatres. So nurses have no or less knowledge about these equipments and their usage.

Future Challenges in Neuronursing

Current literatures in neuroscience is available in every corner of the world. But the neuronursing is lacking behind in its knowledge. So the leaders in nursing profession has to take up the responsibility of giving current trends to their fellow nurses by:

1. Writing articles in national journals.
2. Writing articles in international journals.
3. Conducting continuing education program and ISE program for nurses.
4. Doing research to form nursing theories in neuroscience nursing.
5. Publishing manuals or handouts according to the changes happening in neuroscience.

2

Review of Anatomy and Physiology of Nervous System

The life depends mainly on respiratory and circulatory systems but the quality of life depends on the nervous system and the endocrine system.

The nervous system is composed of a large number of nerve cells called neuron. A neuron consists of a nerve cell, the processes of nerve cell, axon and dendrites.

Neuroglia constitute around 80 to 85 percent of central nervous system. They include astrocytes, oligodendroglia, microglia and ependymal cells. This nuroglia supports, protects and nourishes the neurons. Primary tumors of CNS usually arise from these cells.

Neurons are responsible for transmitting nerve impulses. They do not become neoplastic. Neurons have a cell body, a single long extension called axon and many short processes called dendrites. The cell body of neuron has nucleus and cytoplasm in it and metabolic activities take place in these parts of the neuron (Fig. 2.1).

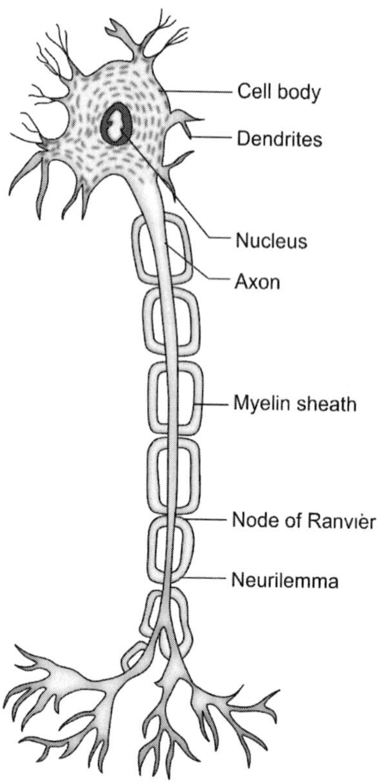

Fig. 2.1: Structure of nerve cell

The axon is a single long process from the cell body of the nerve cell. It has a length which can vary from several micrometers to a meter. The axon is covered by a sheath like structure called myelin sheath. Around the myelin sheath there is thin membrane called neurolemma. At regular intervals the myelin sheath is interrupted and neurolimbia is brought close to the axon cylinder. These constrictions are called Nodes of Ranvier. These nodes are important for the transmission of nerve impulses. The axons as a whole carry the nerve impulses away from the cell body to other organs of the body. The dendrites are short processes which extend from the cell body and receive impulses from the cell axons of other neurons. The structural and functional junctions between two neurons are called synapse (Fig. 2.2).

The end of an axon where the nerve impulse arrives before being transmitted to another neuron is called the presynaptic terminal. The space between the presynaptic terminal and the reception site is called synaptic cleft. When a nerve impulse reaches the presynaptic terminal, it causes the release of chemical substances, which are called neurotransmitters. These neurotransmitters can be excitatory or inhibitory according to the impulse received and the action potential required in each situation. Following are some common neurotransmitters released in CNS (central nervous system).

1. Adrenaline
2. Noradrenaline
3. Serotonin

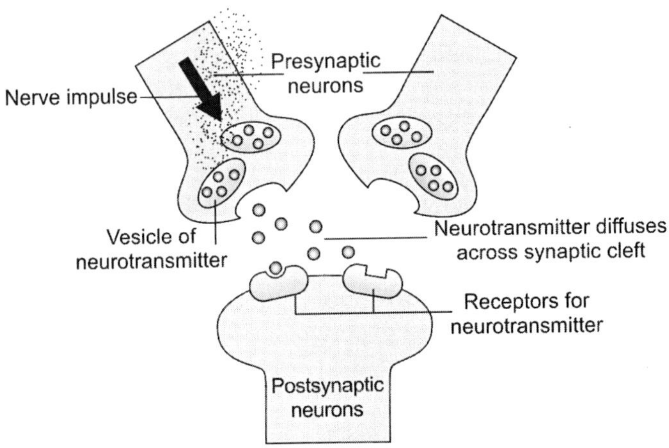

Fig. 2.2: A synapse in nervous system

4. Hydroxytryptamine
5. Gamma aminobutyric acid (GABA).

Any imbalance (alteration) in the production or usage of these neurotransmitters can cause behavioral changes in individuals.

The drugs are composed and dispensed to regulate the mechanism wherein the behavior of the human individual can be modified.

The Membranes Covering the Brain and Spinal Cord

The meninges cover the whole brain and spinal cord. The meninges has three different layers called:

- Dura mater—Outer covering
- Arachnoid mater—Middle layer
- Pia mater—Inner lining.

The Dura Mater

This consists of two layers of dense fibrous tissue. The outer layer lines the skull bones and inner layer covers the brain. These two layers are closely adherent except where the inner layer separates.

1. Cerebral hemisphere—the falx cerebri
2. Cerebellar hemisphere—the falx cerebellar
3. Cerebrum and cerebellum—tentorium cerebelli

It continues beyond the spinal cord (L1,2) and merges with periosteum of coccyx.

The Arachnoid Mater

This is a serous membrane between dura and pia mater—the space between dura and arachnoid mater is called subdural space, through which the cerebrospinal fluid flows. The arachnoid mater continues to envelope spinal cord and ends by merging with dura mater at the level of 2nd sacral vertebrae.

The Pia Mater

This is a vascular membrane. It closely invests the brain completely covering the convolutions and deepening down into each fissure. Beyond the end of the cord, it continues as filum terminal. This filum terminal pierces the arachnoid and dural tubes and goes on to fuse with the periosteum of coccyx.

The Ventricles of the Brain

In the brain there are four irregular shaped cavities, which are called ventricles of the brain. They are named as: the right and left lateral ventricles, 3rd ventricle and 4th ventricle (Fig. 2.3).

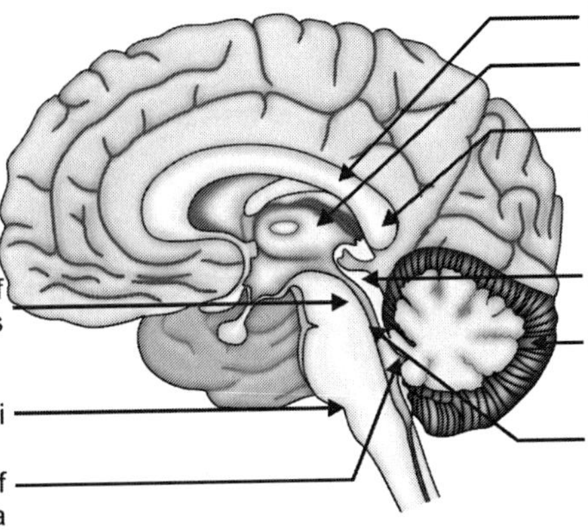

Fig. 2.3: Ventricles of the brain

The lateral ventricles lie within the cerebral hemisphere, one on either side of the median plane just below the corpus callosum. Within the walls of these ventricles, there is highly vascular fringe of membrane called choroid plexus. These ventricles are connected to 3rd ventricles by foramen of Monro. The third ventricle is situated below the lateral ventricles and between the two thalami. The third ventricle is opening to the 4th ventricle by aqueduct of Sylvius. The 4th ventricle is a lozenge-shaped cavity, situated below and behind the 3rd ventricle. The 4th ventricle has a median foramen called foramen of Magendie and two lateral foramina of Luschks. Through these foramens, the ventricle communicate to cisterna magna.

The Cerebrospinal Fluid (CSF)

The CSF is formed and secreted by the choroids plexus of the lateral ventricles. It flows to 3rd ventricle through foramen of Monro. From 3rd to 4th ventricle by aqueduct of Sylvius—4th ventricle has a median foramen of Magendie and two lateral foramina of Luschk through which the cerebrospinal escapes to the cisterna magna. From cisterna magna CSF flows around the spinal cord and brain through the subarachnoid space (Fig. 2.4). It is reabsorbed in the arachnoid mater to circulatory system.

Characteristics of CSF

It is clear, slightly alkaline fluid with a specific gravity of 1004 to 1008. It consists of water, amino acids, mineral salts, glucose, few

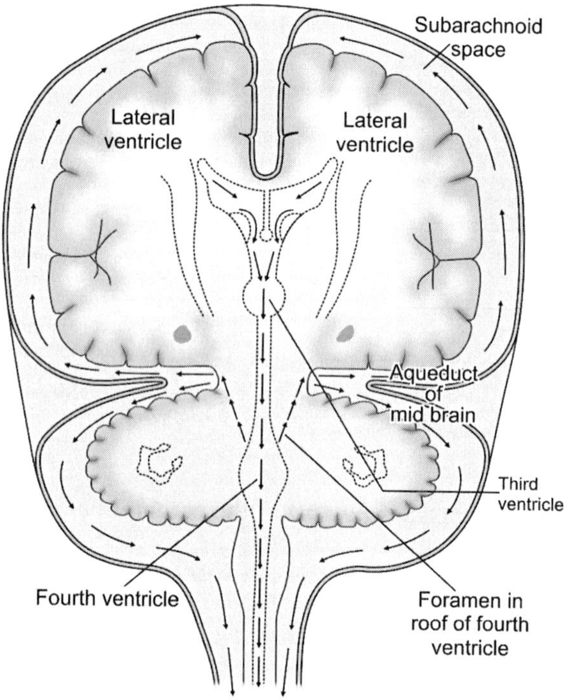

Fig. 2.4: Scheme showing the flow of the cerebrospinal fluid, arrows indicate direction of flow

lymphocytes and some pituitary hormones. The pressure of the fluid may be 70 to 180 mm of water. The quantity present in an adult may vary from 80 to 120-200 ml. This quantity is maintained by the balance between production and absorption.

Central Nervous System

This consists of the brain, spinal cord, peripheral nerves and cranial nerves.

The brain: It constitutes, one-fifth of the body weight and it lies in a hard bony cage called skull. The structures (Fig. 2.5) forming the brain are:

- The cerebrum or forebrain

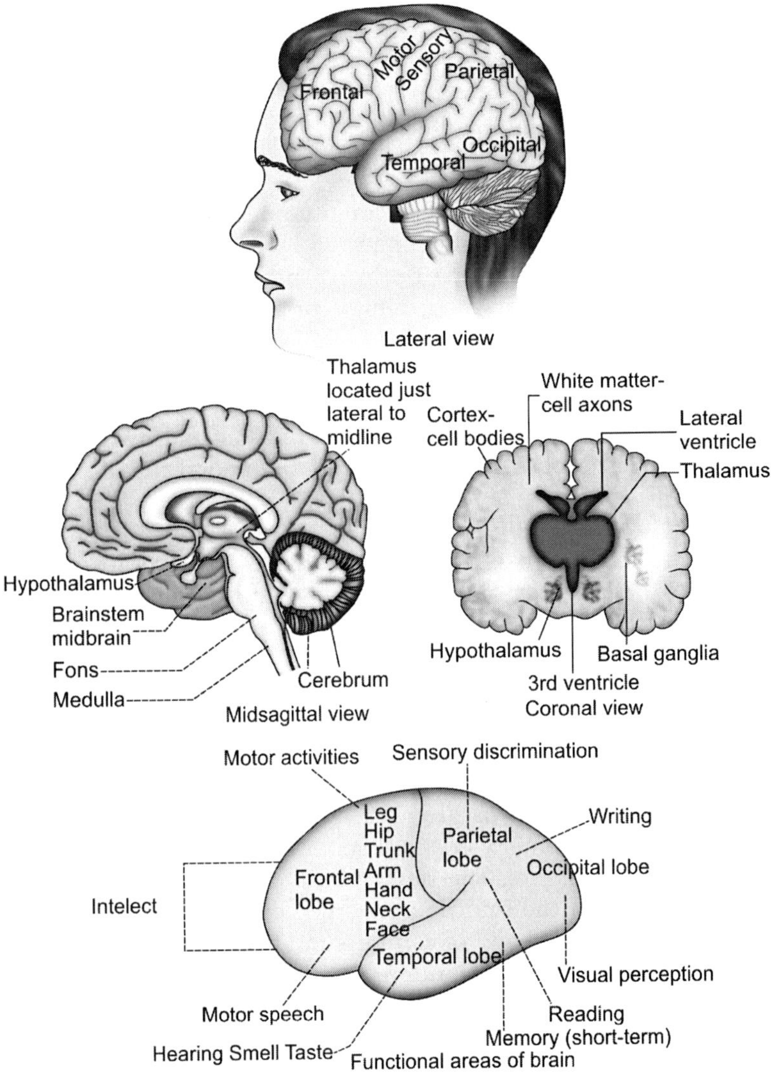

Fig. 2.5: Anatomy of brain—different views

- The midbrain
- Pons varolii
- Medulla oblongata
- Cerebellum.

The brainstem

The hindbrain

The Cerebrum

It is divided into two halves by a longitudinal fissure as right and left. These hemispheres are connected by a mass called corpus callosum. The peripheral part of cerebrum is composed of gray matter forming cortex. The cerebral cortex has many folds, the lapsed areas of folds are called gyri and furrow between the folds are called sulci or fissure.

Each hemisphere of cerebrum is divided into lobes. They have been named to the corresponding bones of the skull under which they are situated. The lobes are frontal, parietal, temporal and occipital.

Functions of Cerebrum

1. Mental activities like memory, intelligence, sense of responsibility, thinking, reasoning, moral sense and learning.
2. Sensory perception—of pain, temperature, touch, light, hearing, taste, smell.
3. The initiation and control of voluntary muscular contraction.

Cerebral Fissures

There are five important fissures which are landmarks.

1. *Longitudinal, cerebral fissure*
   The cerebral hemispheres are separated by a deep vertical longitudinal fissure. The separation is complete in front and behind but in the middle portion, it extends to the corpus callosum, a wide band of commissural fibers, which unite the hemispheres. In the posterior region the cerebrum overlaps the thalamus, midbrain and cerebellum. A process of dura mater extends down into this fissure and separates the two cerebral hemisphere. It is called falx cerebri.
2. *Transverse fissure*
   Transverse fissure is between the cerebrum and cerebellum. The process of dura mater also extends into this fissure and covers the upper surface of the cerebellum and the undersurface of the cerebrum. It is called tentorium cerebelli.

3. *Cerebral sulcus or fissure of Rolando*—Located in between the frontal and parietal lobe on either side.
4. *Lateral cerebral fissure or fissure of Sylvius*—Located between the lower part of the frontal lobe and temporal lobes of cerebrum on either sides.
5. *Parieto-occipital fissure*—Located between parietal and occipital lobe.

Basal Ganglia, Thalamus and Hypothalamus

These are a group of nerve cells situated deep inside the cerebral hemispheres.

The basal ganglia—Influences the skeletal muscle tone.

Thalamus—Receives the impulses of pain, temperature, pressure and touch, in their crude form.

Hypothalamus—Controls the secretions of hormones, concerns with hunger, thirst, control of body temperature, defence reactions like anger and rage.

The Midbrain

It lies between the cerebrum above and pons varolii below. It has two peduncles. It acts as relay station for ascending and descending nerve fibers. The group of cells for transmission of nerve impulses from optic nerve and vestibular portions of the auditory nerve play a major role in the maintenance of balance of body.

Pons Varolii

This is situated in front of cerebellum below the midbrain and above the medulla oblongata. It forms the bridge between the two hemispheres of the cerebellum.

Medulla Oblongata

It extends from the pons varolii above and is continuous with the spinal cord below. It is pyramidal in shape with apex below and base above.

Several important cranial nerves arise from the nuclei in the medulla. The important centers in the medulla are :

- Cardiac center
- Respiratory center
- Vasomotor center
- Reflex centers of vomiting, coughing, sneezing and swallowing.

Cerebellum

It is situated behind the pons varolii and below the cerebrum and lies in the posterior cranial fossa. In cerebellum the gray matter forms the cerebellum and white matter lies deeply. It has three groups of peduncles:

- Superior peduncles
- Middle peduncles
- Inferior peduncles.

Functions

- Muscular tone
- Muscular movement
- Body balance and equilibrium.

Spinal Cord

Spinal cord is the elongated, almost cylindrical part of the central nervous system. It lies within the neural canal of the vertebral column (Fig. 2.6A). It is continuous above with the medulla oblongata and extends from the upper border of the atlas to the lower border of the 1st lumbar vertebra. It is 45 cm (18″) in length and is about the thickness of a little finger.

It is surrounded by three layers of meninges, i.e. dura, arachnoid and pia mater. Subarachnoid space around the spinal cord is filled with CSF as it is around the brain.

Structure of Spinal Cord

The spinal cord is the nervous tissue, linking between the brain and the organs of the body. Nerves conveying impulses from the brain to the various organs of the body descend through the spinal cord. At the appropriate level they leave the cord and pass to the organs which they supply. Similarly sensory nerves from the sensory organs enter and pass upwards to the spinal cord, then to the brain.

Thirty-one pairs of nerves arise from spinal cord, which are called spinal nerve (Figs 2.6B and C). They are named according to the part of neural canal from which they emerge.

The lumbar, sacral, and coccygeal nerve leave the spinal cord before its termination at the level of 1st lumbar vertebrae and extends vertically downwards to occupy the subarachnoid space below this level. They form a sheath of nerves which resembles a horse's tail and is called 'cauda equina'.

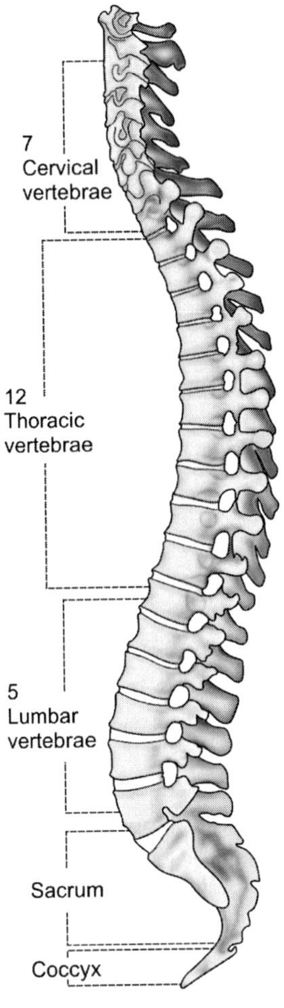

Fig. 2.6A: Vertebral column

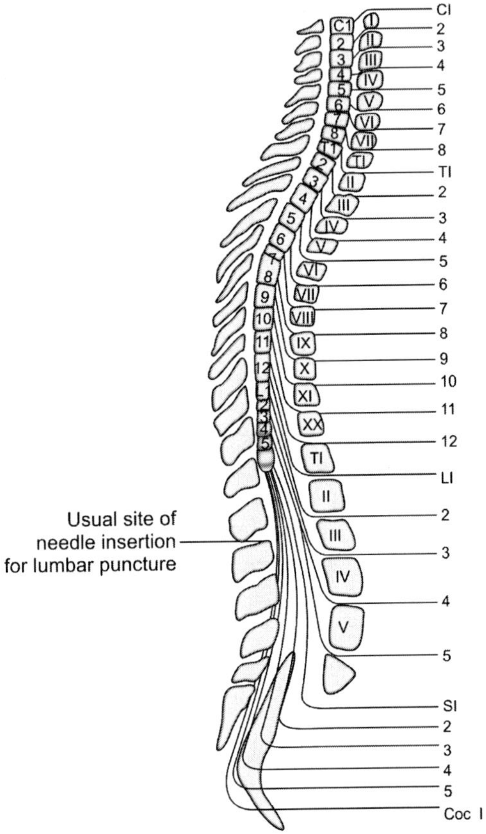

Fig. 2.6B: Position of spinal nerves

The spinal cord is incompletely divided into two equal parts, anteriorly by a sheet, shallow, median fissure and posteriorly by a deep narrow septum known as the posterior median septum (Fig. 2.7).

Reflex Action

Reflex action can be described as an automatic motor response to a sensory stimulus without the brain being involved.

There are a number of familiar reflex actions, e.g.

1. The quick closing of eyelids if the eye is touched, called corneal reflex.
2. Quick recovery of the balance of the body to prevent falling after a slip.

These responses to sensory stimuli are instant although the individual is eventually conscious of their occurrence. A reflex action can only take place if there is a complex reflex arc.

A simple reflex arc (Fig. 2.8) has following three components:

1. Sensory neurons which comprise the sensory nerve endings in an organ, a sensory nerve, the postroot ganglion cell and its nerve fiber which passes to the posterior horn of gray matter in the spinal cord.
2. A connector neuron which consists of nerve cell, its dendrites and axon in the spinal cord.

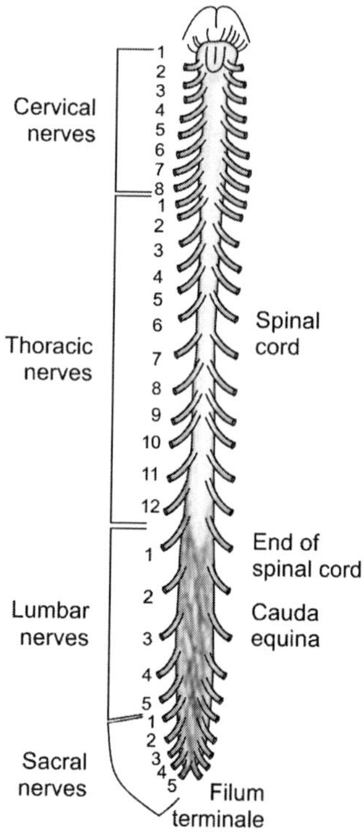

Fig. 2.6C: Anterior view of spinal cord with origination of spinal nerves

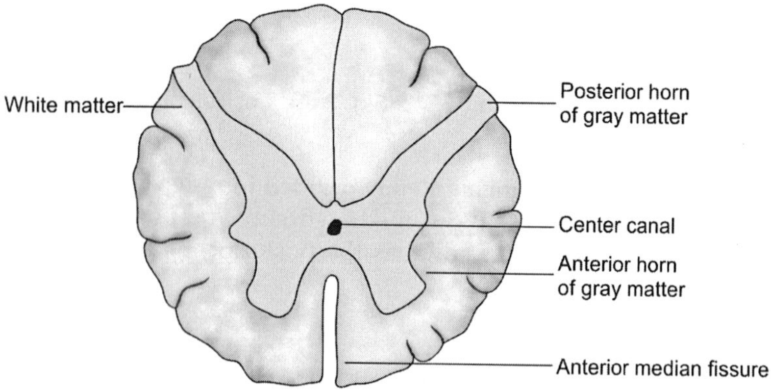

Fig. 2.7: Cross section of spinal cord

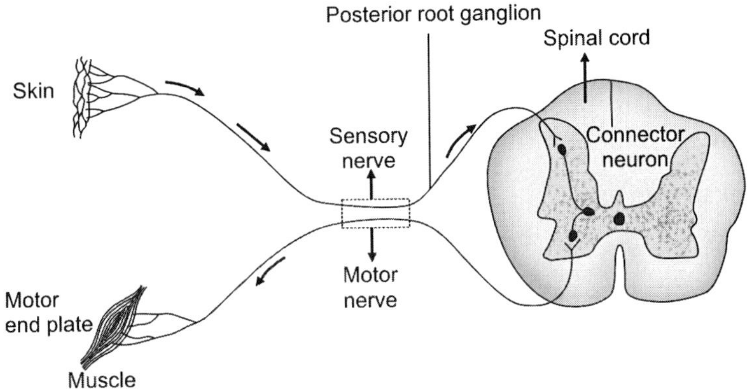

Fig. 2.8: Reflex arc

3. A motor neuron consisting of a nerve cell and its dendrites in the anterior horn of gray matter, the axon of this nerve cell and the motor end plates which terminate in muscle.

Physiology of Reflex Action

The process of reflex action commences when a sensory nerve end is excited or stimulated. The impulse is carried to the spinal cord through a sensory nerve. The sensory neuron which is involved in this, forms a synapse with the dendrites of the connector neuron. The connector neuron may transmit the impulse to the motor neuron at the same level or to a number of motor neurons at different level, depending on the muscles involved in the motor response. A second synapse also occurs where the impulse passes from the connector neuron to the dendrites of the motor neuron. The motor neuron will then convey the impulse to the muscles thus stimulating them to contract.

Reflex actions are carried out so rapidly, even the brain is not directly involved. In infants micturation and defecation are the examples of such action. But as the child grows older, the sensory nerve tracts of spinal cord become fully developed, the impulse from the bladder and rectum reach the brain and can be controlled.

Peripheral Nerves

The peripheral nerves are composed of sensory nerve fibers conveying impulses from sensory end organs, such as skin, eye and ear to the brain, and motor nerves emerging impulses from the brain through the spinal cord to the effector organs, for example skeletal muscles.

The peripheral nerves include 31 pairs of spinal nerves which arise from the spinal cord and 12 pairs of cranial nerves which arise from the brain.

Spinal Nerves

They are 31 pairs in number. They are numbered according to the level of the spinal column from which they emerge. They are grouped and named according to the vertebrae with which they are associated.

- 8 cervical nerves
- 12 thoracic nerves
- 5 lumbar nerves
- 5 sacral nerves and
- 1 coccygeal nerve.

The spinal nerves arise from both sides of the spinal cord and emerge through the intervertebral foramina. Each nerve is formed by the union of motor and sensory nerve roots and is therefore a mixed nerve.

There are five large plexuses formed on each side of the vertebral column. They are:

1. The cervical plexus,
2. The brachial plexus,
3. The lumbar plexus,
4. The sacral plexus, and
5. The coccygeal plexus.

The Cranial Nerves

There are 12 pairs of cranial nerves. They arise directly from the brain. Some of them are sensory, some others are motor and still some others are mixed. They are:

- Olfactory—sensory
- Optic—sensory
- Oculomotor—motor
- Trochlear—motor
- Trigeminal—mixed
- Abducens—motor
- Facial—motor
- Auditory—sensory

- Glossopharyngeal—mixed
- Vagus—mixed
- Accessory—motor
- Hypoglossal—motor.

Cranial nerves central origin, distribution and functions are shown in Table 2.1.

Autonomic Nervous System

Autonomic or involuntary part of nervous system controls the functions of the body which are carried out automatically. These functions do not reach consciousness under normal condition, e.g. rate and force of heart beat, movements of alimentary tract, etc.

The efferent nerves of the autonomic nervous system arise from nerve cells in the brain. These emerge at various levels between the midbrain and the sacral region of the spinal cord. For anatomical and physiological convenience the autonomic nervous system is described in two parts as sympathetic and parasympathetic.

Sympathetic Nervous System—Structure

Three neurons are involved in conveying impulses from their origin in hypothalamus and the medulla oblongata to the effector organs and the tissues:

1. The cell is in the brain and its fiber in the spinal cord.
2. The cell is in the lateral horn of gray matter in the spinal cord, between the levels of the 1st thoracic and the 5th lumbar vertebrae. The fiber of the cell leaves the cord by the anterior root and terminates in a ganglion outside the spinal cord. This fiber is known as preganglionic fiber.
3. The cell is in one of the ganglia and its fiber conveys the impulse to the effector organ or tissue. This is the postganglionic fiber. This is usually longer than the preganglionic fiber.

Parasympathetic Nervous System—Structure

Parasympathetic nervous system is referred as craniosacral outflow of the autonomic nervous system. Two neurons are involved in the transmission of the impulses from their source to the effector organ.

Table 2.1: Cranial nerves: origin, distribution and functions

Name and no.	*Central origin*	*Distribution*	*Function*
1. Olfactory (sensory)	Smell area in temporal lobe of cerebrum through olfactory bulb	Mucous membrane in roof of nose	Sense of smell
2. Optic (sensory)	Sight area in occipital lobe of cerebrum, cerebellum	Retina of the eye	Sense of sight balance
3. Oculomotor (motor)	Nerve cells near the floor of the aqueduct of the midbrain	Superior, interior and medial rectus muscles, and circular muscle fibers of the iris	Moving the eyeball, regulating the size of the pupils and focusing
4. Trochlear (motor)	Nerve cells near floor of aqueduct of midbrain	Superior oblique muscles of the eyes	Movement of the eyeball
5. Trigeminal (mixed)	Motor fibers from the pons varolii sensory fibers from the trigeminal ganglion	Muscles of mastication Sensory to gums, cheeks, lower jaw, iris, cornea	Chewing Sensation from the face
6. Abducens (motor)	Floor of fourth ventricle	Lateral rectus muscles of the eye	Movement of the eye
7. Facial (mixed)	Pons varolii	Sensory fibers to the tongue Motor fibers to the muscles of the face	Sensation of taste Movements of facial expression
8. Auditory (sensory)	Hearing area of cerebrum	Organ of Corti in the cochlea	Sense of hearing

Contd...

Table 2.1 contd...

Name and no.	*Central origin*	*Distribution*	*Function*
9. Glossopharyngeal	Medulla oblongata	Back of tongue and pharynx Posterior third of tongue Parotid glands	Sense of taste Secretion of saliva Movements of pharynx
10. Vagus (mixed)	Medulla oblongata	Pharynx, larynx, lungs, heart, gallbladder, stomach, small and large intestine	Movement and secretion
11. Accessory (Motor)	Medulla oblongata	Sternomastoid, trapezius, laryngeal and pharyngeal muscles	Movement of the head and shoulders and pharynx and larynx
12. Hypoglossal (motor)	Medulla oblongata	Tongue	Movement of tongue

The Cranial Outflow

The preganglionic fiber arises from nerve cells situated in the midbrain, pons varolii and medulla oblongata. Then travels towards ganglia situated in the walls of the organs to be innervated. Postganglionic fibers pass to the muscles or cells to be stimulated.

The vagus nerves are the most important nerves of the cranial outflow.

The Sacral Outflow

The nerves of the sacral outflow pass out with the second, third and fourth sacral nerves from the spinal cord. The preganglionic fibers travel with the pelvic nerves to the ganglia situated near or in the organs to be innervated. The postganglionic fibers then proceed to stimulate the organs.

Functions of the Autonomic Nervous System

The function of the autonomic nervous system as a whole is to adjust and regulate the internal environment of the body. It is responsible for controlling the processes which take place within the body not under conscious control.

It regulates the activities of cardiac muscle, all smooth muscle tissue and glandular tissue. Therefore, glands such as the liver, spleen, salivary glands, gastric and intestinal glands come under its control.

The majority of organs are innervated by both sympathetic and parasympathetic nerve fibers and the effect of one counteracts the effect of the other. *Normally,* they are very delicately balanced, for example, in the control of the size of the pupil of the eye.

Blood Supply to the Brain

The brain receives approximately 15 percent of total resting cardiac output. This figure remains relatively constant because of various control systems affecting the brain. Blood flow rates to specific areas of brain correlate directly to the metabolism of the cerebral tissue. The brain is supplied by two pairs of arteries.

The vertebral arteries arise from the subclavian arteries and ascend on either side and enter the skull through the foramen magnum. The vertebral arteries unite at the level of the pans to become basilar artery. This basilar artery divides again to become posterior cerebral arteries to supply part of the brain.

Mainly the vertebral arteries and their branches supply the cerebellum, the brainstem, the spinal cord, the occipital lobes, the medial and inferior surfaces of the temporal lobes.

The internal carotid arteries originate from two different vessels, the left common carotid which originates directly from aorta, and the right common carotid, which arises from the innominate artery which originates from aorta. The internal carotid artery enters the cranial cavity through the foramen lacerum.

Circle of Willis

The vertebral artery and the internal carotid arteries which enter the cranial cavity along with posterior and anterior communicating arteries to make a circle at the base of the skull. This is called "Circle of Willis" which is responsible for the blood supply of the whole brain (Fig. 2.9).

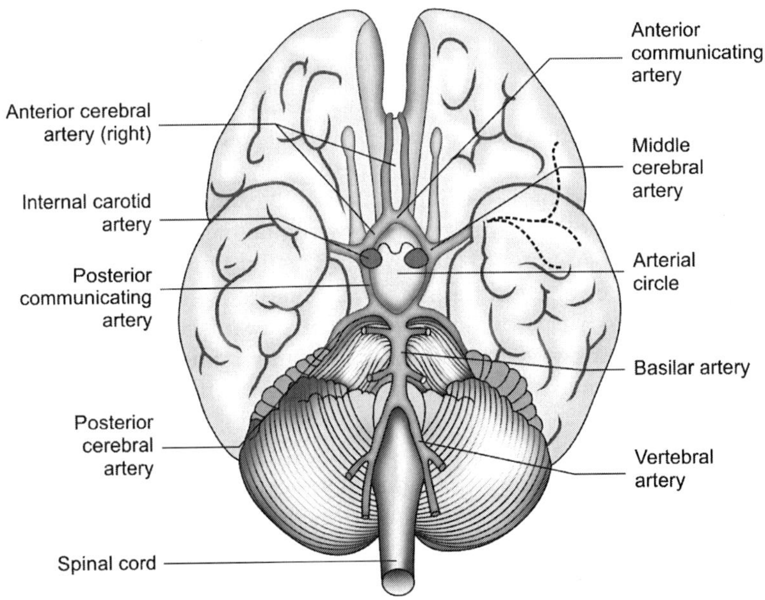

Fig. 2.9: Circle of Willis

The circle of Willis enclose a small area of 6 cm^2. The circle of Willis has a protective mechanism by which the blood was shunted to compensate for alterations in cerebral blood flow or pressure.

Venous Drainage

Venous drainage has a different pattern unlike in other parts of the body which closely follow the arterial pattern. The cerebral venous drainage is chiefly managed by vascular channels created by two dural layers called dural sinuses. There are no valves in dural sinuses. Cerebral veins empty into the dural sinuses which in turn empty into jugular veins which return the blood to the heart.

Blood Supply to Spinal Cord, Spinal Root and Spinal Nerves

The blood supply to spinal cord is from anterior spinal artery and two posterior spinal artery which arise from vertebral arteries. Venous system of the spine includes an intradural and extradural veins follow the pattern of the arteries and extradural intravertebral veins form a plexus extending from the cranium to pelvis. This system has many communications along the way with veins of the neck, thorax and abdomen.

The Blood-Brain Barrier and the Blood Cerebrospinal Fluid Barrier

For the normal function of the central nervous system, a very stable environment in the body is necessary. The so called blood-brain barrier and blood CSF barrier provide that stability for the nervous system. The blood-brain barrier is a descriptive term for the network of capillary endothelial cells and the astroglial membranes located in close approximation to the neuron. The tight junction between the endothelial cells and the astroglial cells are responsible for the barrier. This barrier provides selectivity to the substances that cross the neural membrane and gain entrance into the neuron. Because of this barrier many drugs are prevented from affecting the brain and spinal cord.

The movement of the substances into brain depends on particle size, lipid solubility, chemical dissociation and the protein binding potential of the drug. The drugs that are lipid soluble and undissociated at body pH will rapidly enter both the brain and CSF. The blood-CSF barrier is similar to the blood-brain barrier. Its anatomical structures are found in the choroid plexus.

LIMBIC SYSTEM

The anatomical connections of the limbic system are extremely complex and their significance is not fully understood. The results of neurophysiological experiments, which have included

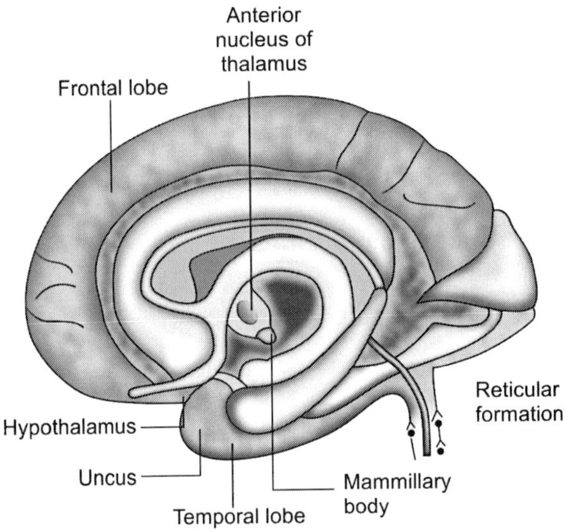

Fig. 2.10: Few connections of limbic system

stimulation and ablation of different parts of the limbic system in animals are not entirely clear.

The word limbic means border or margin and the term limbic system was loosely used to include a group of structures that lies in the border zone between the cerebral cortex and the hypothalamus.

Anatomically the limbic structures include subcollosal, the angulate, the parahippocampal gyri, the hippocampal formation, amygdaloid nucleus, the mammillary bodies and anterior thalamic nucleus (Fig. 2.10). The alveus, fimbria, the fornix, the mammillo-thalamic tract, and the stria terminates constitute the connecting pathways of this system.

Hippocampal Formation

Hippocampal formation consists of hippocampus, the definite gyrus and parahippocampal gyrus.

The hippocampus is a curved elevation of gray matter that extends throughout the entire length of the floor of inferior horn of the lateral ventricle. The thin layer of white matter which lies on the convex ventricular surface is called alveus. The alveus has nerve fibers, which converge medially to form fimbria.

The dentate gyrus is a narrow notched band of gray matter that lies between the fimbria of the hippocampus and the parahippocampal gyrus.

Amygdaloid nucleus—It is so called because it resembles an almond. It is situated partly anterior and partly superior to the tip of the inferior horn of the lateral ventricle. It is fused with the tip of tail of caudate nucleus.

The hippocampus has six afferent connections and efferent connection to function in different directions for different function of the body.

Functions of Limbic System

- Control the endocrine system
- Control emotional behaviors especially fear, anger and emotions related to sexual behavior
- Converting recent memories to long-term memories
- Effective homeostatic responses to a wide variety of environmental stimuli
- Elevation and depression of arterial blood pressure
- Peristalsis of bowel
- Pupillary reaction
- Salivation, chewing, licking
- Bladder contraction
- Sudden attention or surprise
- Grooming.

As the limbic system is responsible for emotions and thinking, any change in limbic system causes symptom of schizophrenia like delusions, auditory hallucination, and even blunted affect.

Research may bring forth much more information about structures and functions of limbic system in coming years.

3

Neurological Examination—Nurses' Role

The neurologic examination provides critical intimation that no other test can provide. It tells us whether the patient's nervous system is working normally or not. It also helps to diagnose and localize the disease within the nervous system.

Purposes of Neurological Examination

Following are the purposes of neurological examination:

1. Nursing purpose of the examination is to determine whether nervous system dysfunction is present or not ?
2. It helps in collecting data that differentiates medical practice from nursing practice.
3. As a part of patients' record, it is available for the nurse and other health professionals for review.
4. Comprehensive neurological examination helps to diagnose the disease and then treatment and nursing can be prescribed accordingly.

In most of the hospitals neurological examination is done by the physician. But it is a duty of the nurse to do some of the neuro -logical examination at the time of admission, and every 4-hour or every 15 to 20 minutes thereafter as per the condition of the patient.

All nurses working with neurological and neurosurgical patients should have the knowledge of neurological examination and should have the skill of assessing the patients for neurological deficits.

Components of Neurological Examination

Following are the components of neurological examination:

1. Level of consciousness
2. Mental status examination

3. Cranial nerve function
4. Motor power
5. Sensory function
6. Cerebellar functions.

Level of Consciousness

The first part of neurological assessment deals with assessing the patient's level of consciousness. Is the patient alert, lethargic, stupor or comatose? The patient's responses should fit into one of the following categories.

- *Alert:* Patient is awake, responds immediately and appropriately to all verbal stimuli.

- *Lethargic:* Patient is drowsy and inattentive but arouses easily. Frequently drops-off to sleep. Cooperates when awake. When the patient is aroused, he is oriented to person, place and time.

- *Stuporous:* Patient spends much of time sleeping. He arouses with great difficulty and cooperates minimally when stimulated, inappropriate responses to verbal commands are evident.

- *Semicomatose:* Patient has lost his ability to respond to verbal stimuli. There is some responses to painful stimuli. Little motor function is seen. When the patient is stimulated with pain nonpurposeful motor activity is seen.

- *Comatose:* When the patient is stimulated there is no response to verbal or painful stimuli. No motor activity is seen.

Mental Status Examination

During conversation note his facial expression, asymmetry or any other abnormal movements. Quality of speech and determine the presence of dysarthria, dysphonia or dysphasia. General intellectual level as well as the activity pattern should be assessed. In addition the following categories should be addressed :

1. *Attention span:* This can be evaluated by patients' ability to repeat a series of five or six digits backward and forward.
2. *Orientation:* Determine whether the patient is able to correctly state his name, the date, including month, year and approximate time of the day and the name of the health facility (time, place and person) and where he is in.
3. *Memory:* Patient's recent and remote memory can be assessed during history-taking.

- Ask the patient to state his date of birth and age.
- Ask the patient to recall mutually known event that occurred earlier in the day.
- Immediate recall can be assessed by requesting the patient to recall three objects told to him three minutes earlier.

4. *General knowledge:* Ask the patient 3 or 4 outstanding items of current events. Assess his knowledge of the present or past names of the ministers. The questions can be planned according to the patient's education level.
5. *Mood and behavior:* Note the patient's general reaction to his illness and the appropriateness of his behavior. Observe the patient for anxious, excited, depressed or paranoid responses to questions.
6. *Appearance:* The attire and grooming and personal appearance of the patient should be appropriate for his age. A neat and clean appearance reflects good grooming and good personal hygiene habits. An unkempt appearance on the other hand might indicate depression or chronic organic brain disease.

Assessment of Cranial Nerves

Each cranial nerve is examined systematically.

Olfactory: Olfactory (I) cranial nerve controls the sense of smell. This test is not required in routine purpose. However, if the patient has sustained a traumatic injury to the face or head, the nurse should test for the function of the nerve. To assess the sense of smell instruct the patient to

1. close the eyes,
2. occlude one nostril, and
3. identify the odor.

Repeat using the opposite nostril.

During the test patient is requested to smell and identify benign substances such as coffee, cloves, lemon or soap. Strong pungent odors such as alcohol, acetone and ammonia which may irritate the patients mucosa should not be used.

Optic Nerve (II): Second cranial nerve controls visual activity and the visual field. To assess visual activity:

1. Instruct the patient to cover one eye.
2. Position a magazine or newspaper 12 to 18 inches from the patient.
3. Instruct the patient to read at different levels of print.

Gross visual activity may also be assessed by having the patient count fingers by closing one eye and repeat using the opposite eye.

Gross assessment of visual field is determined by confrontation. The patient should be instructed to cover one eye. The examiner closes her/his opposite eye. The examiner then positions her fingers off to the side at eye level at the same distance between the patient and herself. The examiners' moving finger is, then brought into the main boundaries of the visual field. The patient states when the moving finger is seen. This exercise is repeated with patient using her opposite eye.

Fundoscopic examination: Fundus is examined by looking through the pupil with ophthalmoscope. Retina, retinal arteries, veins and optic nerve head are seen. Increased ICP is manifested by congestion of vein and swelling of optic nerve head (papilloedema).

Oculomotor (III), Trochlear (IV) and Abducens (VI) cranial nerves:

Oculomotor (III) cranial nerve controls pupillary reaction. The three nerves oculomotor, trochlear and abducens cranial nerves function together to control extra oculomovements.

Pupillary reaction is assessed by:

1. Instructing the patient to fix his eyes on an object.
2. Shining the beam of open light or flashlight directly into each pupil.
3. Noting the size, shape and reaction of the pupils to the light stimulus. The pupil size should be noted before and after the light is directed into the eye.

To assess ocular movement ask the patient to follow an object moved systematically in various direction—up, down to the right and to the left and should note for the presence of diplopia, limited eye movement and the presence or absence of nystagmus.

Trigeminal (V) cranial nerve: The trigeminal *(V)* cranial nerve has both sensory and motor components and controls facial sensation and jaw movements.

To assess the sensory function of this nerve, patient should be asked to close his eyes, then the various parts of face is gently touched using a wisp of cotton. The patient is asked to identify where the cotton is applied each time.

Motor function of this nerve is evaluated by telling the patient to open her/his mouth wide and hold tightly. Then examiner attempts to close the patient's mouth using hands.

Facial VII cranial nerve: The facial, VII cranial nerve has both motor and sensory functions. The nerve controls the facial muscles and supplies taste fibres to the anterior two-third of the tongue. Assessment of taste function is not routinely performed. Motor function is assessed by having the patient wrinkle her forehead, smile, showing her teeth and wink her eyes. Asymmetrical movement or facial drooping to be noted.

Auditory or Acoustic (VIII) cranial nerve: The acoustic, VIII cranial nerve controls hearing and the sense of balance.

Hearing can be tested by using a ticking watch one to two inches away from the patient's ear or using a tuning fork, hearing in both the left and right ears should be compared. Whispering can also be used to test hearing.

The Weber test and Rinne test may be done to differentiate between conduction deafness and nerve deafness. Weber test is used to evaluate lateralization. Whereas the Rinne test evaluates air and bone conduction. Abnormal results warrant further investigation.

Glossopharyngeal (IX) and Vagus (X) nerves: Glossopharyngeal (IX) and vagus (X) cranial nerves control swallowing, the gag reflex, articulation, and phonation. To assess these functions:

1. Instruct the patient to open his mouth and say 'ah'; normally the soft palate and uvula elevate in the midline, if there is paralysis, uvula deviates to side.
2. Use the tip of a tongue depressor, very gently, stimulate the back of the pharynx. Any asymmetrical contractions of the palate uvula and pharynx are noted.
3. Swallowing is tested by asking the patient drink a clear fluid and noting the reaction.

Spinal accessory (XI) cranial nerve: The spinal accessory (XI) cranial nerve controls the trapezius and sternocleidomastoid muscle. These muscles assist the patient in shoulder shrugging and head and neck movements.

1. To assess trapezius muscle function, instruct the patient to raise both shoulders and to hold tightly and apply resistance to both shoulders using hands.
2. Sternocleidomastoid muscle function is evaluated by asking the patient to turn her/his head against resistance applied by using hands of the examiner.

Hypoglossal (XII) nerve: The hypoglossal nerve controls tongue movement and strength. This function is appraised by having the patient protrude her tongue. Normally it protrudes in the midline. To assess tongue strength, instruct the patient to move her tongue to the right and to the left.

Assessment of Motor Function

For routine determination of muscle strength, a few simple tests are usually sufficient. As with all other aspects of the assessment meticulous comparison must be made in symmetry with each side of the body. Both distal and proximal muscles of the arms and legs must be tested.

When assessing the distal and proximal muscle strength of the upper and lower extremities, the following guidelines to be used :

1. To assess the motor function, apply maximum force to the extremity while the patient pushes against the observer's fixed resistance.
2. Grade the motor function according to the guidelines in the chart below.
3. Use the following abbreviations when referring to each extremities.
    - D-Distal
    - P-Proximal
    - RUE-right upper extremity
    - RLE-right lower extremity
    - LUE-left upper extremity
    - LLE-left lower extremity.

Motor power gradings:

Grade	*Description*
5/5	Full range of motion against gravity with extreme resistance
4/5	Full range of motion against gravity with some resistance
3/5	Full range of motion against gravity, no resistance
2/5	Full range of motion with gravity eliminated
1/5	Slight contraction visible
0/5	No movement.

After assessing muscle strength of the upper and lower extremities, the arm and leg drift test to be tested. To test the arm drift, request the patient to close her eyes.

The patient is instructed to extend her arms with palms facing upward.

The position should be maintained for 10 seconds.

Note any upward or downward drift of the arms.

To test the leg drift, ask the patient to close the eyes. The patient is instructed to hold both legs out in front while sitting on the edge of the bed. This position should be maintained for 10 seconds. Note any upward and downward drift of the legs.

Assessment of Sensory Functions

Basic assessment of sensation includes investigation of the patient's bilateral response to touch, pain, temperature and position sense.

- Response to touch can be evaluated by using a wisp of cotton to gently touch various parts of the patient's body. Ask the patient identify where the sensation is felt with each tactile stimulation.
- To assess the patient response to pain, use a sterile 22 gauge needle or a safety pin which has been cleansed with alcohol to gently touch various parts of the patient body. Request that the patient identify where the sensation is felt.
- Temperature response is assessed by using two clean test tubes, one filled with warm water and one filled with cracked ice. Various parts of the patient's body are gently touched with each tube. The patient is asked to distinguish between hot and cold touch on various parts of her body.
- To assess the patient's position sense, instruct the patient to close her eyes and then grasp the patient's index finger at the last joint from the side and gently raise or lower it.
- The patient is asked whether the index finger is positioned up or down. This exercise is repeated using the patient's great toe.

Assessment of Cerebellar Functions

For routine purposes, the finger to finger, finger to nose, Romberg, tandem walking and patting tests provide adequate information for evaluation of balance and coordination.

- *Finger to finger test:* It is performed by instructing the patient to place her index finger in the nurses index finger. She is asked to repeat this maneuver several times in succession on both sides.

- *Finger to nose test:* To perform the finger to nose test, tell the patient to extend her index finger and then touch the tip of her nose several times in rapid succession. This test is done with the patient's eyes open and again with the eyes closed.
- *Patting test:* Patting test is administered by asking the patient to hold her hands and arms above her thighs with palms positioned downward. She is then told to slap her thighs simultaneously. The patient is then requested to raise her hands above her thighs, turning her hands over and again slapping her thighs. These actions are repeated several times in rapid succession.
- *Romberg test:* To perform the Romberg test, instruct the patient to stand with her feet together with arms positioned at her sides. She is told to close her eyes. This position is maintained for 10 seconds. The Romberg test is considered positive only if there is actual loss of balance.
- *Tandem walking test:* It is tested by having the patient assume a normal standing position. She is then instructed to walk, heel to toe on a straight line. Any unsteadiness, lurching or broadening of the gait bone is noted.

Role of the Nurse during the Examination

The role of the nurse is to be supportive of the patient, providing brief explanations, emotional support, and physical support as necessary.

The usual equipment necessary to conduct a neurological physical examination includes the following :

- Ophthalmoscope
- Otoscope
- Tongue blade
- Tuning forks
- Pin
- Tape measure
- Flash light
- Reflex hammer
- Wisp cotton
- Small containers having:
  Salt, pepper, coffee powder, soap, lime, etc.
  Two test tubes for hot and cold water.

Nurses' role in assisting the doctors to do the neurological assessment is important. But to do a brief neurological assessment is most important for a nurse in neurowards. Because the nurse in neurowards should have a basic data of the patient for further assessment and act and report immediately if, there is any deterioration at any time of the day or night. So this chapter of this handbook is so vital to a nurse working for patient with neurological or neurosurgical problems.

4

Diagnostic Procedures in Neurological Conditions—Nurses' Role

Diagnostic tests and procedures for the patients with neurological disorders are fewer in number, but more sophisticated than in the past. Computed tomography (CT) and now magnetic resonance imaging (MRI) have revolutionized the armamentaria available for diagnosis of neurological diseases. With the high-tech environment of neuroscience practice, the nurse assumes responsibility, not only for the actual physical and psychological management of patient before and after diagnostic testing but also for patient and family teaching.

Neurological diagnostic procedures are performed in a variety of settings including the radiology department, special procedure areas and patient care unit. Those patients undergoing a diagnostic procedure need a general explanation of the procedure with special emphasis on what to expect and their role as participants. It is the responsibility of the nurse to provide adequate explanation and support to patient and family members.

The various neurological diagnostic procedures are:

1. X-ray
   - Skull
   - Spine
2. Anatomical imaging techniques of the brain
   - CT scan
   - MRI
3. Physiological imaging techniques of the brain
   - Position emission tomography (PET)
4. CSF and spinal procedures:
   - Lumbar puncture

- Myelography
- Lateral C1-C2 puncture
- Ventricular puncture

5. Cerebrovascular studies
   - Cerebral angiography
   - Digital substraction angiography (DSA)
   - Doppler imaging
6. Nervous system electrical activity and conduction
   - Electroencephalography (EEG)
   - Electromyography (EMG)
   - Nerve conduction velocity
   - Evoked potential
7. Testing of special senses
   - Audiometric studies
   - Caloric testing
8. Biopsies
   - Muscle biopsy
   - Nerve biopsy
   - Brain biopsy.

X-ray

X-ray of skull and face:

- View: Anterior, posterior, lateral views
- Special views: View of optic foramen, petrous bones, sellat-urcica, paranasal sinuses.

Purposes

1. To determine the presence of a skull fracture
2. Unusual calcification
3. The size and shape of the bones
4. Bone erosion
5. Abnormal vascularity
6. Presence of air.

Key Points in Understanding Skull Film Reports

1. Fracture through base of the skull or paranasal sinuses may produce pneumoencephalus or air in the temporomandibular joint.

2. A skull fracture with a depression of more than 0·5 cm will result in an underlying contusion.
3. Most depressed skull fractures require surgical debridement.

Nurses' Responsibility

1. Give brief explanation about the procedure and purpose of the procedure.
2. Provide psychological support.
3. Put hospital uniform or cotton dress.
4. Encourage the patient to lie still for few moments necessary to take films.

Spinal X-ray

Spinal X-rays are simple X-rays of various regions of the spine : cervical, thoracic, lumbar or sacral.

View : Anterior, posterior and lateral views are most commonly taken.

Indication

1. Trauma to the back or vertebral column.
2. Conditions in which the patient experiences pain, motor or sensory impairment.

Abnormal Findings

Various abnormal findings may include :

1. Wedging of a collapsed vertebra
2. Erosion of bone
3. Irregular calcification (osteophyte, spur)
4. Narrowing of the vertebral canal
5. Vertebral fracture and dislocation
6. Spondylosis.

Nurses' Responsibility

1. Explain briefly the procedure and the purpose of it.
2. Provide necessary emotional support.
3. Put hospital uniform or cotton dress.

ANATOMICAL IMAGING TECHNIQUES OF THE BRAIN

CT Scan (Computed Tomography)

CT scans were initially introduced for the use in clinical diagnosis by Hounsfield in England in 1972. Now it represents the cornerstone of neurological diagnostic procedures. This technological advance has been accepted for its accuracy, safety and versatility for use in all body systems.

During the CT scan, the head is scanned in successive layers by narrow X-ray beams that pass through head and are absorbed and transmitted, depending on the density of the tissue. The thickness of a scanner layer, called a slice can vary from 1.5 to 10 mm. Slices are taken at a slightly angled horizontal plane. Recent spiral scanners can reconstruct images even at 0.8 mm.

The radiation transmitted from the tissue is detected by an array of scientillation crystals (scanner) that converts the transmitted X-ray (radiation) into light photons in proportion to the energy and intensity of the transmitted radiation. The photons are, in turn converted to electrical signals that are digitized and the information can be manipulated by specialized computer programs to reproduce images representing the various slices of the cranium/ brain in various orientations. (Coronal, sagittal, horizontal) on a display monitor. The display image may be photographed with standard X-ray or polaroid film.

The digitized conversion of the images results in anatomical visualization which correlates to tissue density. The denser structure:

- Bones appear as relatively whiter areas.
- CSF and air are less dense, therefore appear as black areas.
- Brain parenchyma appears as various shades of gray.

Procedure

The patient lies on an X-ray table, with face uncovered and head immobilized. A movable circular frame encircles the head and revolves around it making a claking sound while taking radiographic readings. The head is scanned numerous times at different angles. If contrast medium is injected to enhance certain areas, additional pictures are taken after a short delay. The entire procedure lasts for 15 to 30 minutes and the patient has to remain motionless as movement can cause artifacts within the image that will affect the clarity of the picture. However, a spiral scanner can perform the entire examination in less than a minute and thus can be used to scan uncooperative patients.

Indications

a. CT scan is extremely useful in localizing and diagnosing various cranial lesions, such as abscesses, cysts, infarctions, hematomas, contusions, hydrocephalus and primary and secondary metastatic tumors.
b. To identify ventricular size.

Advantages

a. It is a painless and safe procedure.
b. Much information can be collected when a problem is still in its early stages.
c. Cost is relatively reasonable and drastically reduces the need for more invasive diagnostic tests such as cerebral angiogram.
d. It can be performed on both conscious and unconscious patients.
e. Radiation exposure is relatively low compared to that of skull films.
f. Serial CT scans can be taken to follow the resolution of cerebral disorders (hemorrhage, edema, etc.)

Disadvantages

a. It has decreased sensitivity in detecting lesion adjacent to bone, soft tissue lesions.
b. Uses radiation.

Nurses' Responsibility

1. A nurse should give a general explanation of the procedure and the equipment used to prepare the patient psychologically.
2. Consent to be taken and patients should be told that they must remain very still while the scan is being taken to ensure accuracy and quality graphs.
3. All jewellery, eye glasses and metal objects shall be removed from the head.
4. No dietary restrictions if contrast is not given.

5. If contrast is planned
   - keep the patient nothing per mouth for 4-5 hours before the test.
   - find out if patient is asthmatic or is allergic to any drugs.
6. For children and restless patients, sedation may be given. (For children phenergan syrup or trychloryl syrup; for adults injection serenace 5-10 mg usually given).
7. For some children or adults who are not cooperating or having involuntary movements, CT may be done under general anesthesia.

During the Procedure

1. Before radiopaque contrast medium is administered, a skin test to be done to check for allergic reactions.
2. While giving contrast patient is asked to take deep breathing till the injection is completed.

Postprocedure

1. Observe the patient who received contrast medium for delayed allergic reaction such as hives, skin rash, itching, nausea, headache, swelling of face, breathlessness.
2. If symptoms are severe antihistamines and hydrocortisone may be given as per the hospital policy. (Usually avil 1-2 ml and hydrocortisone 100 mg IV is given.)
3. Patient should be hydrated to clear contrast from the body, faster.
4. Patient who had CT under general anesthesia is kept on IV fluids and nothing per mouth for a few hours.

MRI (Magnetic Resonance Imaging)

Magnetic resonance imaging (MRI) provides greater resolution and detail than does CT, but takes longer to perform. Because it uses a powerful magnetic field, there is no exposure to radiation.

Procedure

MRI is noninvasive, painless procedure and carries no known risk to the patient. After removing all metal objects, the patient lies on a padded stretcher that slides into a tunnel like chamber. The head is placed in a plastic helmet like structure. The arms are at the side of the body and are held in place with velcrostraps. The head of the

X-ray table is then rolled several feet into the scanner. The patient is placed in a strong magnetic field up to 40,000 times stronger than the Earth's magnetic field and is then subjected to precise, compute programmed bursts of radiofrequency (RF) waves. The patient feels nothing and hears only loud noises caused by the pulsating RF waves that resemble a jackhammer or drill which lasts about a few minutes.

Advantages of MRI over CT

a. Provide detailed images for precise lesion assessment, and localization.
b. No harmful effects of radiation.
c. It gives not only anatomical information but also information about the chemistry and physiology of living tissue.
d. It gives multiplanar images. (can imagine any plane without changing the position of the patient).
e. Can study blood vessels without the administration of contrast media.
f. Provides higher resolution detail of the posterior fossa, skull base and orbits as compared to CT scan.
g. It is excellent in detecting soft tissue changes like necrotic tissues, oxygen deprived tissues, small malignant tumors, degenerative diseases, ischemic areas, hemorrhage and arteriovenus malformations, etc.

Disadvantages

a. Expensive.
b. Relatively not available.
c. Contraindicated in patient with metallic devices such as artificial pacemakers, prosthetic devices, (metallic hip replacements, orthopedic pins) artificial limbs, etc.
d. Not possible in uncooperative patients and those with claustrophobia who cannot tolerate the closeness of the tube to their face.
e. Cannot reliably detect calcification.

Nursing Care

1. Patient should be told that it is a painless procedure and he/she will hear a lot of noises during the procedure and it is necessary to remain still for upto 45 minutes in very close quarters.

2. All jewellery, eye glasses and hairpins/clips or any other metal objects should be removed. Carefully question and screen for the presence of any metal implantation.
3. Consent for contrast and for general anesthesia to be taken.
4. Patient should wear only cotton dress.
5. No dietary restriction for MRI even for contrast, unless anesthesia is planned.
6. Extra blanket may be provided as the patient is in the AC for more than 45 minutes.
7. During the procedure when contrast is needed, first 1 ml is given very slowly to observe for any reaction.

Postprocedure Care

1. For patient who had MRI under general anesthesia kept fasting for 3 to 4 hours and IV fluids to be given.

Comparison of indications for CT scan and MRI

CT scan	*MRI*
• Pacemaker in place*	• Allergy to contrast medium
• Metal prosthesis in place*	• Subacute/chronic cerebral trauma
• Uncooperative patients*	• Pituitary tumors
• Acute craniocerebral trauma	• Posterior fossa lesions
or acute intracerebral hemorrhage	• Demyelinating diseases (multiple sclerosis)
• Aneurysm clipping with metal*	• Cerebral atrophy
• Hemorrhagic stroke	• Spinal cord trauma
• Hydrocephalus	• Intervertebral disk diseases when myelographic results are normal

*MRI contraindicated

PHYSIOLOGICAL IMAGING TECHNIQUES OF THE BRAIN

PETT (Positron Emission Transaxial Tomography)

Positron emission transaxial tomography (PETT) is a noninvasive technique that is useful in studying biochemical and physiological function in a living organism such as glucose uptake and metabolism, O_2 uptake and cerebral blood flow pattern.

Principle

The technology is based on the use of an online cyclotron (electromagnetic machine) and positron emitting radionuclides are created.

The patient inhales or is injected with a compound that has been labelled with a positron emitting nuclide 'tag' (often carbon 11) once inside the body, the compound selected concentrates in the area of clinical interest and emits positrons that reacts with electrons producing gamma rays of specific energy. A special scanner detects the gamma rays and encodes the data into a computer which reconstructs cross-sectional images of the tissue containing the labelled compound.

Indications

PETT is a new, developing technology used primarily for studying complex physiologic process. It is used in CNS research to improve the understanding of—epilepsy, dementia, (e.g. Alzheimer's disease) cerebrovascular disease, cerebral trauma and mental illness.

Procedure

After 6 to 12 hours of NPO (nil per mouth), the patient is placed on a stretcher in the imaging center and prepared. An arterial line may be inserted to draw blood samples for measurement of cerebral metabolic rate. The radio pharmaceutical agent of choice is injected via venous access. The patient rests quietly in a dimly lighted room for about 45 minutes while uptake of the drug occurs. Only head is placed inside the scanner. If blood sample is required, it is drawn quietly without disturbing the environment. The scanning procedure takes 45 minutes. The entire procedure takes about 2 to 3 hours.

Advantage

Images through the procedure are very clear in comparison to the conventional radionuclide scans.

Disadvantages

a. It is an expensive study.
b. Online cyclotron equipment is found only in a few major research centers.
c. It is used for diagnostic purposes for only a limited number of patients.

Nurses' Role

1. Maintain NPO for 6 to 12 hours before the procedure.
2. No glucose solution, intravenous infusions should be used.
3. After completion of the study, fluids should be encouraged to clear the radioisotopes from the body.

Cerebrospinal Fluid (CSF) AND SPINAL PROCEDURES

Lumbar Puncture (LP)

Definition

Introduction of a hollow needle with a stylet into the lumbar subarachnoid space of the spinal canal using strict aseptic technique.

Purpose

The reason for doing a LP may be diagnostic or therapeutic.

Diagnostic

1. To measure the CSF pressure.
2. To obtain CSF for visualization and laboratory examination.
3. To inject air, oxygen or radiopaque substance to visualize parts of nervous system.
4. For evaluation of spinal dynamics for signs of blockage of CSF flow due to tumor or other pathology of spinal cord.

Therapeutic

1. To remove blood or pus from subarachnoid space.
2. To reduce intracranial pressure (ICP).
3. To give spinal anesthesia for surgeries.
4. For intrathecal injection of antebacterial and other drugs.

Contraindication

1. Cutaneous or osseous infection at the site of the lumbar puncture.
2. When paticnt has drastically increased ICP, lumbar puncture may result in brain stem compression, and "coning" through foramen magnum and ultimately death.

Procedure

The LP is usually done at patients bedside or in an outpatient facility. An LP set is prepared. Patient assumes a lateral recumbent position along the edge of the bed arching the back, so that the knees are flexed on the chest, with the chin touching the knees. This position allows maximal separation of the vertebrae thereby facilitating insertion of LP needle and reducing degree of trauma. Prepare the site aseptically, drape and locally anesthetized. Strict aseptic procedures to be followed. Place the needle between L3 and L4 or L4 and L5. After introduction, the stylet is removed and a manometer is affixed to measure and record the entrance pressure of CSF. Then manometer is removed and samples of CSF are collected into sterile test tubes for visual and laboratory examination. When procedure is completed, LP needle is removed and a band-aid is applied over the puncture site.

Complications

1. Trauma to the tissue at the LP site.
2. Headache.
3. Infection.
4. Injury to spinal cord and spinal nerves.
5. Local pain edema and hematoma at the puncture site.
6. Herniation or coning of brain through foramen magnum.

Nurses' Responsibility

1. Ask the patient to empty the bladder immediately before the procedure.
2. Briefly explain the procedure and purpose of the procedure and provide emotional support.
3. Informed consent to be taken.
4. Privacy during the procedure to be provided.

Postprocedural Care

1. Patient should be kept in prone position 2 to 3 hours following the procedure.
2. Foot end of the bed should be elevated.
3. Frequently monitor neurological and vital signs.
4. Patient may have headache due to irritation of brain/mild analgesics may be given according to hospital policy.

Table 4.1: Characteristics of cerebrospinal fluid (CSF)

	Parameter	*Normal value*	*Abnormal finding*
1.	Volume	About 135-150 ml	Volume increased with hydrocephalus Decreased in space occupying lesions
2.	Specific gravity	1.007	Increased with blood cells and infection
3.	Color	Crystal clear	Discoloration (xanthochromia) looks red in intracranial hemorrhage and traumatic hemorrhage – Turbidity indicates an increased number of WBC – Clouding indicates increased protein content or microorganisms
4.	Protein	15-45 mg/100 ml	Increased with tumors, infections and hemorrhages
5.	White blood cell	0-5 cells/mm^3	10-200 cells mostly lymphocytes occurs in viral meningitis, multiple sclerosis, tumor and neurosyphilis
6.	Glucose	40-80 mg/100 ml (approx. 80%)	Decreased in glucose indicates presence of glycolytic substances such as bacteria in the CSF
7.	Pressure	76-200 mmH_2O	Increased in intracranial pressures

Myelography

Definition

It is a diagnostic procedure ordered to visualize the lumbar, thoracic or cervical areas or whole spinal axes for diagnosis of a spinal tumor, a herniated intervertebral disk or a ruptured disk.

Indications

1. To diagnose spinal cord tumor
2. To visualize herniated intervertebral disks
3. To find out a ruptured disk.

Procedure

An LP is performed and approximately 10 ml of CSF is removed. Water soluble nonionic contrast medium (maximum 10 ml) is then injected into the subarachnoid space and X-ray films are taken of the spinal cord and vertebral column. Once the water-based contrast medium is injected into CSF, it diffuses upward through the CSF and penetrates into nerve root sleeves, nerve rootlets and narrow areas of the subarachnoid space. The head is kept elevated about 30 degree at all times and the patient is kept quiet. By minimal changes in position of the table and patient, various regions of the spine are screened and films taken at appropriate levels.

Nurses' Responsibility

1. Patient should be well-hydrated.
2. No food prior to myelogram.
3. Procedure to be explained and psychological support to be given.
4. Explain that patient should take more fluids (3 L) first 24 hours after the procedure.
5. Written consent to be taken.

Postprocedural Care

1. Keep the patient on bedrest for 4 hours with head elevated 30 degrees.
2. Should be kept quiet and still for 24 hours.
3. Encourage more oral fluids.
4. Monitor neurological and vital signs.
5. After 4 hours diet to be given if no nausea or vomitings.
6. Mild analgesics may be given if headache persists.

Lateral C1-C2 Puncture

Definition

Introduction of a short bevelled needle with a stylet in the lateral subarachnoid space between C1 and C2.

Indications

1. To remove CSF for laboratory analysis when impossible to obtain it at the lumbar level.
2. To demonstrate subarachnoid block by doing a cisternal puncture simultaneously with LP.
3. To introduce radiopaque or air for myelography.
4. For therapeutic drainage if a lumbar puncture is contraindicated or if a subarachnoid block is present, below the level of C1-C2.

Nurses' Responsibilities

Preparations

- Explain the procedure and purpose to the patient.

- Get written consent.
- Shave the nape of neck up to the occipital protrubarence.
- Skin to be prepared as if for surgical operation.

Position

Patient lies on one side with the head in neutral position and held firmly by the nurse.

Procedure

After preparation of the skin and after giving local anesthesia, a needle is inserted just beneath the base of the skull to a depth of about 5 cm. The needle is very close to medulla, so great care is required in positioning, steadying and reassuring the patient.

Postprocedure Care

- Patient should be watched for cyanosis, dyspnea and apnea.

Ventricular Puncture

Definition

Insertion of a needle into lateral ventricle. In infants a short beveled No. 22 needle with a stylet is introduced through scalp into the anterior fontanel. In adults a ventricular needle is directed through an opening in the skull made with a burr or trephine.

Indications

- If LP and cisternal punctures are unsuccessful or contra-indicated.
- For injection of dye into the ventricles of an infant to determine the type of hydrocephalus present.
- To remove fluid quickly after ventriculography or craniotomy if the patient shows evidence of increased ICP.
- To inject air or oxygen directly into ventricles for localization of a tumor when encephalography is contraindicated.

Nurses' Responsibility

- Get a written consent.
- Give sedative for infants if necessary.
- Anterior one-third of head is shaved and cleaned with soap and water.

- Keep ready tapping set or twist drill set.
- Give emotional support to the patient and family.

Postprocedural Care

- Watch the patient closely.
- Check for signs of collapse or increased ICP.
- Monitor vital signs and level of consciousness.
- Place the patient on his side with head elevated.
- If continuous ventricular drainage is placed it should be maintained under a septic precautions.
- Ventricular drainage to be observed for free drainage; if there is any block, immediate care to be taken.

Complications

- Fever, hemorrhage, infection, oozing of CSF from wound, and meningitis are the common problems of this procedure.

CEREBROVASCULAR STUDIES

Cerebral Angiography

Definition

Cerebral angiography is the X-ray study of the cerebral circulation following injection of contrast material into a selected artery.

Indications

a. To visualize the cerebral arteries and veins to determine the size and site and nature of pathological process.
b. To locate the tumors, abscesses, aneurysms, hematomas or other lesions large enough to distort grossly the normal cerebral vascular pattern and to study the pattern of blood supply.
c. As a preparatory investigation to neurovascular interventional therapy.

Contraindication

- Severe kidney, liver or thyroid disease.
- History of an allergy to the contrast material.

Procedure

The patient is placed in a supine position on the X-ray strecher. A wide area around the puncture site, usually groins is shaved and cleaned. A local anesthetic is usually administered (2% xylocain). After local injection, the contrast medium is injected directly into the carotid artery or introduced by the indirect route, through catheterization of carotid or vertebral arteries using femoral, brachial, subclavian or axillary arteries. X-ray films are then taken at various time intervals for visualization of the intracranial and extracranial blood vessels. When the test is completed direct manual pressure is applied to the puncture site for 5 to 10 minutes to prevent bleeding into subarachnoid space.

Complications

- Allergic reactions to contrast media, seizures, stroke, pulmonary emboli, thrombosis, symptoms of carotid sinus sensitivity (hypotensions, syncope).

Nurses' Responsibility

Preparations

- Patient to be prepared psychologically.
- Skin to be shaved at puncture site, for direct puncture. In male patient, beard and neck to be shaved. For transfemoral approach shaving to be done for both male and females from umbilicus to mid thigh on both sides.
- A consent form outlining the risks to be signed by the patient.
- Patient should be told to lie still during the procedure and he will feel a burning sensation during the injection for 4 to 6 seconds.
- For female patient indwelling catheter and for males urocondom to be fixed.
- Patient should be given regular antihypertensive, antiepileptic and other drugs.
- Nil by mouth to be observed for 6 to 8 hours for the patient posted under general anesthesia.
- Mark the appropriate peripheral pulses with a felt tipped pen on the skin.

During the Procedure

- The nurse in the angiogram room will receive the patient, explain the procedure, reassure the patient and place the patient on the table.
- Legs and hands are fixed.
- Blood pressure (BP) cuff and EEG leads are applied and connected to the monitor and IV is started.

- Xylocain test dose is given.
- Painting and draping is done for femoral artery puncture.
- Heparin injection is given after the puncture, according to the needed dosage. Injection heparin is given every hourly.
- Vital signs are checked continuously.
- At the end of the procedure, heparin is neutralized by giving protamine injection.
- Pressure crape bandage is applied to the puncture site after ensuring no bleeding in the puncture site, then peripheral pulse is felt and patient is shifted to the ward.

Postprocedure

- Nurse in the ward checks the pedal pulse and puncture site for hematoma and bleeding.
- Patient should put on complete bed rest for 12 hours.
- If the puncture site is femoral artery, the leg is immobilized for 24 hours to prevent bleeding.
- Observe puncture site frequently for bleeding and check the color and temperature of the extremity.
- If there is bleeding at the puncture site, pressure bandage to be applied and the concerned doctor to be informed immediately.
- Monitor vital signs and neurological signs.
- Encourage more fluids to clear the contrast.
- Remove the plaster at the puncture site only after 24 hours.

Digital Subtraction Angiography (DSA)

Definition

DSA is a computer assisted radiographic procedure for visualization of the carotids and other cerebral vessels. The image produced is made more distinct by the elimination of surrounding and interfering anatomical structures. This is accomplished by recording images before and after injection of contrast medium and subtracting the first image from the second.

Indications

1. The purpose of DSA includes assistance in the diagnosis of the following conditions:
   - Atherosclerotic disease (stenosis, occlusion, ulcerations)
   - Vascular lesions. (AV malformation, aneurysms, carotid cavernous fistular)

- Postoperative evaluation of endarterectomy, aneurysm clipping, arteriovenous malformations, repair and anastomosis.

2. It is done for interventional radiology.

Procedure

Selected vessels are visualized with an image—intensifier that displays vessels on a monitor. Pictures are taken and stored on a magnetic tape. The images which are collected by the computer before contrast injection are received and then subtracted from those taken after injection. So that the image of the desired area is enhanced. The remaining contrast—enhanced images can be manipulated by the computer to focus on specific problems that might otherwise not be visualized. After completion of the procedure, the catheter is removed. Pressure is applied to the puncture site for several minutes and sterile dressing is applied. The whole procedure may take 30 to 45 minutes.

Nursing responsibilities are same as done for cerebral angiogram.

Doppler Imaging

Definition

Doppler imaging is a noninvasive diagnostic method for vascular study.

Procedure

It is a procedure in which a Doppler ultrasonic probe (which sends high frequency sound waves) is placed in the skin over the vessel in accessible region/part.

The sound waves strike the moving red blood cells within the lumen of the blood vessel and the sound reflected back to the Doppler probe represents the velocity of the blood flow. These data are amplified and a graphic recording and sound recording of the blood flow are produced.

The test is safe noninvasive method with high accuracy. It takes 15 to 45 minutes to complete.

Purpose of Doppler in Neuroradiology

Carotid artery
- Atherosclerotic arterial occlusion
- Stenosis
- Aneurysm

Vertebral artery
- Stenosis/block
- Reversal of flow

Jugular vein
- Thrombosis/occlusion
- Recanalisation after occlusion.

Nurses' Responsibilities

1. The patient should be explained about the procedure which is painless.
2. Patient should be instructed to remain still during the procedure.

NERVOUS SYSTEM ELECTRICAL ACTIVITY AND CONDUCTION

Electroencephalography (EEG)

Definition

EEG consists of graphic records of electrical activity of the brain, using multiple scalp electrodes. It provides physiologic assessment of cerebral activity.

Indications

- To diagnose the epilepsies.
- Used as a screening procedure for coma and organic brain syndrome.
- Indicator of brain death.

Procedure

The patient quietly lies with eyes closed. Electrodes are arranged on the scalp to record the electrical activity in various regions of the brain. The amplified activity of the neurons is recorded on a continuously moving paper sheet. This record is the encephalogram.

Nurses' Responsibility

- Nurse should explain the procedure and ensure patient cooperation.
- Reassure the patient that he will not receive an electric shock and it is a painless procedure.
- Withhold the medications such as anticonvulsants, stimulants, tranquilizers and depressants for 24 to 48 hours, because that can alter the brain wave activity.
- Coffee, tea, colas and chocolates are withheld in meal before test because of their stimulant effect.
- Thorough hairwash with soap or shampoo to be given.
- No oil to be applied after the bath.
- Patient should be put on only cotton dress.
- Should have good breakfast half to one hour before EEG.

Postprocedure Care

- The hair is washed to remove the electrode affixing paste.
- Any drugs that were withheld specifically for EEG are resumed.

Electromyography

Definition

Electromyography is the recording of muscle activity at rest, during voluntary movement and with electrical stimulation are made by inserting small needle electrode into the muscle.

Indications

1. To help in the diagnosis of myasthenia gravis.
2. To find out peripheral nerve injury or disease.
3. To find out whether primary problem is in nerve or muscle.
4. To differentiate among lesions of the anterior horn cell, root, plexus and specific nerve and muscle.

Procedure

The procedure is performed by inserting a needle electrode into a muscle and analyzing motor unit potentials both at rest and in varying degrees of muscle contraction.

Nurses' Role

- Explain the procedure and ensure cooperation from the patient.
- Patient should have good breakfast half to one hour before the test.
- Patient should wear only cotton dress (terylene, nylon clothes to be avoided).

Nerve Conduction Velocity Studies

Definition

Nerve conduction velocity studies measure the conduction time and amplitude of electrical stimulation along two or more points of peripheral nerve using a cathode (negative electrode) and an anode (positive electrode).

Peripheral nerve is stimulated at several points along its course and its muscle action potential and sensory action potential is recorded.

Indication

Helpful in diagnosis of neuropathies induced by diabetes, alcoholics, nutritional deficiencies, compression or trauma to peripheral nerves.

Nurses' Role

- Explain the purpose and procedure of the test to the patient.
- Provide psychological support to the patient.

Evoke Potential

Definition

Evoke potentials is a recording of electrical activity in central sensory pathways produced by visual, auditory or sensory stimulation. Signals are recorded by placing electrodes over the scalp or the spine and using a computer to average and amplify the signal which results in characteristic pattern of wave from peaks that have approximate anatomic correlates. There are three types of evoked potential studies.

- Visual evoked responses (VER)
- Brainstem auditory evoked responses (BAER)
- Somatosensory evoked potentials (SSEP).

Indications

- Used in the diagnosis of multiple sclerosis.
- Brainstem lesions are verified and localized by BAER.
- Acoustic neuroma (BAER used to verify CN8 injury).
- Spinal cord injury (SSEP differentiates completely from partial injury).
- Hypoxic coma (Absence of cortical potentials by SSEP implies that conscious will not be regained).

Nurses' Role

- Explain the procedure and provide emotional support.
- Head should be washed with soap or shampoo.
- Do not apply oil over the head after the bath.
- Provide good breakfast one hour before evoked potentials.
- Put on only cotton clothes.

TESTING SPECIAL SENSES

Audiometric Studies

Definition

It is a test to assess the auditory branch of the eighth cranial nerve for type and cause of hearing loss. Testing is devided into pure tone audiometry and speech audiometry.

Hearing loss in neuroscience patients is usually related to head injury, meningitis, acoustic neuroma or drug toxicity.

Caloric Testing

Definition

Caloric testing is a diagnostic procedure designed to evaluate the vestibular position of the eighth cranial nerve. The underlying principle is that thermal stimulation of the vestibular apparatus with cold water will elicit the oculovestibular reflex. The test is contraindicated in patients with a ruptured tympanic membrane.

Nurses' Responsibility

Preparation

- Nil by mouth for at least 8 hours before procedure.
- Explain the procedure.
- Provide emotional support to the patient.

Postprocedure

Bedrest should be given until nausea, vomiting, dizziness are subsided.

BIOPSIES

Muscle and Nervous Biopsy

The specimens are very fragile, so procedure should be performed by an experienced surgeon. Sural nerve and gastrocnemius muscle are often examined.

— Muscle biopsy is done to diagnose causes of myopathy, it is performed in cases of
  - polymyositis,
  - genetic biochemical deficiency,
  - mitochondrial disease,
  - infections (trichinosis).

— Nerve biopsy is done to diagnose causes of neuropathy, performed in the cases of
  - vasculitus,
  - leprosy,
  - lymphoma,
  - cytomegalovirus,
  - sarcoidosis,
  - amyloidosis.

Nurses' Role

- Explain the procedure and prepare psychologically.
- Keep the biopsy set ready for use.
- Observe for bleeding after the biopsy.
- Daily dressing to be done till it heals completely.

Brain Biopsy

Brain biopsy can be performed either as an open procedure or by using stereotactic needle localization. It is done for diagnosing brain tumors or abscess, central nervous system vasculitis, neurosarcoidosis and encephalitis.

Nurses' Role in Stereotactic Brain Biopsy

- Prepare the patient psychologically.
- Observe for hemorrhage after the test.
- Check for vital signs.
- Ensure that specimen is sent to the lab.

5

Interventional Neuroradiology—Nurses' Role

INTRODUCTION

Informational technology and industrial revolution makes the radiology branch, especially intervention in radiology sophisticated and more advanced one, compared to other branches.

Angiography involves outlining the intracranial and extra-cranial blood vessels to find out any abnormality with the injection of contrast media.

Digital subtraction angiography (DSA) produces a clearer image by abolishing surrounding anatomical structures. This is done by obtaining images before and following injection of contrast media and then subtracting the first image from the second.

The therapy may be curative, palliative or adjunctive to surgery and the route of intervention is endovascular.

The three main interventions performed in neurological and neurosurgical conditions are:

1. Occlusion or embolization of abnormal neurovascular structures
2. Lysis of thrombotic materials
3. Dilatation of stenosis.

I. EMBOLIZATION

Definition

Embolization is the process in which embolic agents are pushed through the microcatheter and the vascular abnormalities are treated temporarily or permanently.

Indications

Five basic types of abnormal vascular structures can be treated by embolization:

1. Fistula (a simple straight tube)
2. AVM (arteriovenous malformation is a network of channels without an interventing fitter).
3. Tumor: A vascular bed with a capillary network.
4. AV fistula
5. Postcapillary venous (cavernous) angioma.

Punctural Sites

- Femoral artery puncture
- Direct carotid artery puncture
- Auxillary artery puncture.

Complications

1. *Deterioration in conscious level:* It may occur due to angio - graphy or anesthesia and it may occur during or after procedure. Any alterations in consciousness should be reported immediately.
2. *Hematoma:* Hematoma at the punctural site is painful and it may occur if the pressure is not applied properly. In carotid puncture, hematoma will compress trachea and cause asphyxiation in which emergency tracheostomy is necessary.
3. *Pneumothorax:* The subclavian artery lies close to the apex of the lungs and the plura may be unintentionally punctured. The patient will be breathless, cyanosed and complain of chest pain, in which case chest drain and intensive physiotherapy is required.
4. *Other complications:*
   - Rupture of aneurysms → death of patient
   - Weakness of limbs
   - Side effects due to contrast
     a. mild—skin rashes, nausea, vomiting, irritation, etc.
     b. severe—myocardial infarction, cardiac arrest, etc.
   - Transient global amnesia and cortical blindness
   - Complication due to anesthesia.

Types of Embolization

Embolization can be divided into:
- Temporary
- Permanent.

Temporary Embolization

In case of tumors (meningiomas), the embolic particles or agents (e.g. PVA, gel, foam, etc.) are pushed through microcatheter in order to reduce the vascularity of the tumor before taking to surgery, so that blood loss during surgery can be reduced.

Permanent Embolization

In case of aneurysms or AVM, the embolic agents (coils or histocryl) are pushed through microcatheter and it can be cured and in case if it is successful surgery is not needed.

Embolic Agents

Embolic agents can be
1. Particulate embolic agents
2. Mechanical embolic agents
3. Liquid embolic agents.

Particulate Embolic Agents

a. *Polyvinyl alcohol particles (PVA)*
   - Sizes vary from 50 to 150, 150 to 250, 250 to 350, 350 to 500, 500 to 750, 750 to 1000 microns diameter and larger.
   - Particles may be permanent, but the occlusion may not be.
   - Initially it make inflammatory reaction which leads to giant cell foreign body structure which further leads to occlusion.

b. *Gelfoam*
   - Gelfoam (gelatin) is used in occlusion of small to medium size vessels.
   - It is used in protection of normal vascular territory by proximal occlusion before particulate.
   - It is temporary because recanalization occur in 7 to 30 days.

c. *Avitene*
   - Sizes vary from 75 to 150 microns.
   - It is a temporary agent.
   - Once penetrated, distally it will cause ischemia, platelet agglutination and granulomates. All these leads to occlusion of vessels.
   - If it is added with ethanol, it will be used for permanent occlusion.

d. *Angiostat*
   - Size is 75 microns.
   - It cause mechanical obstructions and used for small vessels.
   - It is of povine origin.

e. *Autologus clot*
   - It is perfect temporary agent.
   - It is easily lasting for the duration (about an hour) of proximal embolisation when the main trunk is to be protected.

f. *Pulsar particles*
   - They are permanent but recanalisation may occur.
   - Sizes varies from 150 to 1400 microns.
   - Once it is delivered it will become hydrated and swell by 40 percent. Thus it will occlude the vessels.

Mechanical Embolic Agents

a. *Platinum microcoil*
   - It is made up of Dacron fibers which will enhance thrombogenicity.
   - It is MRI compatible and highly fluoroscopic.

b. *Stainless steel coil*
   - It is of macrosize and made up of Dacron fibers which leads to thrombogenicity.
   - It is used for occlusion of large vessels, e.g. Duran sinuses, vein of galen malformation, etc.

c. *GDC*
   - GDC (Guglielmi detachable coil) are made up of platinum microcoils.
   - Sizes vary from 2 mm to 10 mm in diameter and length vary from 2 cms to 30 cm.
   - The coil is detached from its steel shaft by means of electric current passing through the coil.
   - Advantage is it can be withdrawn at any moment if it is not detached by electrolytic process.

d. *Liquid coils*
   - It is made up of extremely fine platinum.
   - It is used in treatment of AVM in conjunction with cynocrylates.

- It reduce the flow rate (blood) through the AVM before embolization with glue.

e. *Detachable balloons and nondetachable balloons*
- It is made up of latex or silicone.
- Signs varies from 1 mm to 3 mm in the deflated form and inflated form approximately any way from 5 mm to 2 cm.
- Silicon balloons are semi permeable.
- Latex balloons are imperable.
- The detachable balloon has got a radiopaque gold tip marker.

Liquid Embolic Agents

a. *Histoacryl*
- It is liquid polymer which solidifies immediately when it comes in contact with saline/blood.
- It comes in sterile flaxone 0.5 mm size.
- The unolock syringes, bowl, needles, gloves etc. to be dry and sterile.
- The only fluid which can be used to wash hands, the hub of microcatheter, the lumen should be 5 percent dextrose.
- Care to be taken avoid spilling of histoacryl on direct contact skin or eye.

b. *Hydroxyethyl methacrylate*
- It is liquid polymerizing agent used inside of a detachable balloon for permanent occlusion.
- Various salient features are
  - i. It will become 100 percent solid if it mix with saline or blood.
  - ii. It does not expand when polymerizing.
  - iii. It is low viscous so that it is easy to inject through micro-catheter.

c. *Dehydrated ethanol*
- It produces cytotoxic reaction in the target organ and sclerosis of the arterial walls which result in thrombosis.
- It is extremely dangerous agent and must be used with caution.

d. *Fibrin glue*
- It is used to embolize facial AVM.
- It is a mixture of autologus cryoprecipitate and thrombin.
- Once it is injected it will form solid fibrin clot.

NURSING ROLE PRIOR, DURING AND POSTPROCEDURE

Nurses' Role Prior to Procedure

- Patient preparation
- Maintenance of equipments
- Sterilization of catheter
- Maintenance of aseptic technique.

Patient Preparation

It includes psychological and physical preparation of the client.

Psychological Preparation

Explain the procedure to the client which includes proposed treatment, risks and alternative treatment.

Check consent whether it is taken from patient and from patient's closest relatives.

Physical Preparation

- Skin preparation—Area of umbilicus to midthigh should be shaved completely without any cuts or abrasions and the area should be cleaned with skin antiseptic lotion.
- Fasting—NPO after midnight before the procedure. (may have oral medications with sips of water especially antiepileptic drugs).
- Investigations—Blood should be sent for serum electrolytes, RBS, urea and creatine other include ECG, CT scan. X-ray, etc.
- Patient should have bath prior to procedures.
- Patient should be catheterized.

Maintenance of Anesthetic Equipments and Drugs

- Check whether laryngoscopes, ventilator, suction, O_2 and N_2O_2 lines are working.
- All sizes of ETT (endotracheal tube) should be kept ready.
- All anesthetic drugs and emergency drugs should be kept ready.
- The area should be well-spotlighted.

Packing and Sterilization of Catheter and Ancillary Equipment

- All types of catheters (diagnostic, guiding catheter, etc.) should be washed and flushed with plain water and they should be soaked in H_2O_2 for 12 hrs. After that they should be washed in plain water and dried without any particles inside the tubes. Later to be packed and sent for gas sterilization.
- Microcatheters should be washed with plain water and later with H_2O_2. Then they should be dried and to be packed with formalin tablets at least 12 hrs prior to procedure.
- All the materials of steel should be washed well and sent for autoclaving.

Maintenance of Aseptic Technique

- Allow only authorized medical personnel in catheter lab.
- Persons entering catheter lab should wear dresses provided and should wear footwear kept in the lab.
- Before and after each procedure catheter lab should be cleaned with aseptic solution.
- At least once in a week fumigation should be done.

Role of Nurse during Procedure

- Receive patients with all documents, i.e. case file, blood investigations, ECG, CT, X-ray, etc.
- Check the vital parameters and examine the patient condition—level of consciousness, whether moves all the limbs, pupillary reaction and whether fit for anesthesia, etc.
- Maintain patient safety and comfort.
- Start and maintain infusion lines.
  - i. For continuous I/V infusion.
  - ii. For rapid fluid administration in case of complications.
- Assist anesthetist in induction if patient is uncooperative or if needed.
- Assist radiologist in order to get ready for procedure.
- Provide angiogram sets and all other sterile equipments.
- O_2 by masks should be administered (3 to 4 liters) if the patient is not intubated.
- Systemic heparinization after sheathing.

i. Once sheath is in artery administer heparin 5000 IU stat and it is followed by 2500 IU hourly.
ii. Obtain PTT value before giving 6th dose of heparin and dose should be adjusted according to value.

- Watch for
  i. Airway pressure
  ii. Breathing pattern
  iii. Level of consciousness
  iv. Monitor for CO_2, SPO_2, ECG waves, mean pressure, etc.
- Keep on watching for any complications related to contrast media, procedure, etc.
- Maintenance of sheath and microcatheter patency by continuous infusion of normal saline by pressure bag.
- Administer medications as per order and ready and act as per situation.
  i. Antibiotic (cefaloxine) should be administered in B/W procedure if there is increased risk of contamination.
  ii. Administer Avil (1 ml) IV and hydrocortisone (100 mg) if any side reaction occurs due to contrast, etc.
  iii. Administer phenytoin if patient had seizures.
- Maintain intake and output chart.
- Maintain nurses record from starting to end of procedures which includes
  i. Patient condition
  ii. Hourly vital chart
  iii. Heparin dose given
  iv. If any sedation given.

Role of Nurse after Procedure

- Heparin should be reversed with protamine sulfate and it should be based on basis of 1 ml, i.e. 10 mg for every 1000 units of IV heparin.
- Assist the anesthetist to extubate if patient is given GA.
- Apply pressure bandage on the puncture site once the bleeding is secured.
- Explain to the patient and patient attender about the importance of keeping the leg straight.
- Check vital parameter and record it.
- Check whether peripheral pulse is felt or not.

- Transfer the patient to ICU or ward depending upon patient's condition with following instructions.
    i. Watch for bleeding or hematoma at the puncture site.
    ii. Immobilize lower limbs for 12 hours.
    iii. Continue IV fluids if not contraindicated.
    iv. Check vital signs every ½ hourly for first 4 hours and afterwards 2 hourly and chart it.
    v. Continue medication as it is if not contraindicated.
    vi. NPO for six hours if the patient is sedated or given GA.
    vii. Total nursing care should be given, i.e. nutritional aspect, comfort, eliminational needs, etc.

These are the various roles of pre, inter and postembolization procedure which a nurse has to play.

II. LYSIS OF THROMBOTIC MATERIALS

Thrombolysis is a procedure by which a blood clot can be lysed, to restore blood supply. This lysis is usually done by administering a pharmaceutical drug (e.g. An enzyme like urokinase) into the clot itself or as proximal to the clot as possible. For the delivery of such agents, microcatheters are used. The clot can be in the venous sinuses or in main arteries supplying the brain.

III. DILATATION OF STENOSIS

Vasodilatation is also an interventional procedure to augment blood supply by transcatheter methods. A catheter with a balloon (e.g. Fogarthy's) is passed endoluminally across the narrowed focal segment of the artery in such a way that the balloon is in approximation with the stricture. The balloon is inflated such that the narrowed arterial segment is stretched circumferentially and the luminal diameter is increased. The balloon is deflated after adequate dilatation is achieved. This is called angioplasty. Furthermore, to prevent restenosis, a metallic stent can be placed within the narrowed segment after angioplasty. The stent is mounted on a microcatheter and placed at the desired site. The stents are currently available for extracranial use only.

Nursing responsibility for thrombolysis and dilatation of stenosis is mostly like in embolization with modification in drugs.

CONCLUSION

As neuro-interventional radiology is advancing, it is important for the nurses to improve their knowledge related to tools and devices to become efficient nurses in neuroscience nursing.

6

Care of the Patient

UNCONSCIOUS PATIENTS

Unconsciousness is a term used widely to denote a state of unresponsiveness of an individual to an external stimuli. It can be a transient feature or it can be with no observable response to even a deep stimuli which is called coma.

Unconsciousness can be defined as a state in which the cerebral functions are decreased, the individual is unresponsive to sensory stimuli.

Causes of Unconsciousness

Trauma

- To the brain
- To any other organ which can cause hypovolemia

Vascular condition

- Cerebral thrombosis
- Cerebral embolism
- Ruptured aneurysm
- Intracranial hemorrhages

Space occupying lesions

- Tumor
- Abscess
- Subdural hematoma
- Severe concussion of brain
- Contusion of brain
- Extradural hematoma

Epilepsy

Systemic conditions

- Uremia
- Diabetes
- Alcoholism
- Over dosage of drugs

Any organic condition in brain
Psychogenic shock: Any unexpected incidents.

Diagnosis

Diagnosis is done by
- History
- Investigations looking for any infection, organic conditions like uremia, diabetes, over dosage of drugs, toxicity.
- X-ray of skull looking for any space occupying lesion.
- CT scan /MRI to localize the space occupying lesion.

Management

- Management can be medical or surgical according to the cause.

Observation

- Observation is done by using Glasgow coma scale which is discussed in a different chapter of this book.

Nursing management is mainly
- Observation for early diagnosis of deterioration of the patient.
- Special nursing care according to the cause of unconsciousness.
- General nursing care to prevent further complications of other systems.

Nursing Care of Unconscious Patients

It can be discussed under following heads:
Maintain airway
- Patient is kept in lateral position.
- Airway is inserted to prevent the tongue from falling.
- Suctioning is done to clear the throat.
- Endotracheal tube is inserted if needed.
- O_2 is administered by mask or through endotracheal tube.
- Artificial ventilator is connected if indicated.
- Tracheotomy is indicated in some conditions.
- Adjust the ventilators and maintain synchrony or asynchrony on respirator.

Observation of vital signs
- Monitor vital signs frequently.
- Document arrhythmias.

- Do not make the patient sit if the blood pressure is low and pulse rate is high.
- Elevate the extremities to prevent local edema.
- Observe and monitor the neurological signs frequently and report if there is any detoriation.

Maintain personal hygiene

- Mouth care to be given at least twice a day.
- Eye care is given at least twice a day.
- Eyes to be protected with pad or with eye ointment to prevent injury and infection.
- Modified bed (water bed) is used to prevent pressure sores
- Body bath is given daily with special care to pubic, axilla and groin.
- Skin care is given frequently by turning the position of patient every 2 hours and giving care to the bony prominents/ dependant areas of the body.
- Hair is to be combed and tied at least everyday.
- Finger nails and toe nails are cut at least weekly.

Provide sufficient nutrition

- Nutrition is taken care by giving tube feeding or IV fluids.

Maintain urinary and bowel movement

- Intake and output chart is maintained.
- Watch for any urinurea, dysuria.
- Watch for incontinence and use condom drainage/urinary catheter.
- Condom/catheter to be changed frequently.
- Clean the area of condom or catheter daily.
- Irrigate the catheter if needed.
- Urine routine investigation is done frequently to look for any infection.
- Avoid constipation.
- Give enough fluids.
- Use suppositories if needed.

Prevention of contractures

- Passive exercises are given to prevent contractures.
- Keep the body in proper alignment to prevent any disuse syndrome.

Special nursing care to be carried out according to the diagnosis, drugs used and surgery if done. Nursing care should also aim at the early rehabilitation of the patient with minimum complication.

PATIENTS WITH INCREASED INTRACRANIAL PRESSURE

Intracranial pressure is the pressure exerted by the cerebrospinal fluid within the brain. Normally the intracranial pressure measures between 80 mm and 180 mm of water or 0 mm to 15 mm of Hg. When it is increased more than 15 mm of Hg, it is considered as abnormally elevated. Intracranial pressure can vary in different locations or compartments of brain. The pressure in tissue adjacent to an expanding space occupying lesion can be elevated but at the same time the intraventricular pressure can be within the normal limits. Increased intracranial pressure may not be consistently conveyed to the lumbar subarachnoid pressure.

The skull is a rigid compartment which is filled with brain matter (80%), intraventricular blood (10%) and cerebrospinal fluid (10%). If any one of these component increase in volume, another component must decrease for the overall volume to remain constant. This will be only on skulls after they are fused.

Before the actual signs and symptoms of increased intracranial pressure are manifested, the contents of brain go through certain compensatory mechanisms. They can be discussed as it is shown in Table 6.1.

Causes of Increased Intracranial Pressure

1. Increased brain volume due to space occupying lesions like hematoma, tumors, abscess aneurysms or cerebral odem.
2. Increased blood volume due to obstruction of venous flow, hyperemia or hypercapnia. Head injuries causing injury to blood vessels bleeding from aneurysms.
3. Increased cerebrospinal fluid due to
   - increased production of CSF by choroid plexus of ventricles.
   - decreased absorpotion of cerebrospinal fluid.
   - or obstruction to the flow of cerebrospinal fluid.

Signs and Symptoms of Increased Intracranial Pressure

The signs and symptoms of increased intracranial pressure are
Early signs

- Confusion, irritation, restlessness and deterioration in the level of consciousness.
- Headache.

Table 6.1: Different stages of increased intracranial pressure and their effects

Stage	*Intracranial pressure*	*Effect*
Stage 1	No increase in intracranial pressure is associated with an expanding mass	Compensation phase, no changes in vital signs
Stage 2	Slight increase in the mass of brain. Results in great elevation of intracranial pressure	End stage of compensation, changes in vital signs are slight to moderate
Stage 3	Intracranial pressure can reach arterial blood pressure	Beginning stage of decompensation, • Deterioration of level of consciousness • Abnormal respiratory patterns • Increased systolic blood pressure • Widened pulse, bradycardia, cardiac arrhythmia
Stage 4	In normal autoregulatory mechanism Fails to increased level of CO_2 by dilating cerebral arteries to supply nutrients and oxygen to brain. If the condition is not treated arterial and intra-cranial pressure becomes equal resulting in the no blood flow and death	Decompensation phase - symptoms noted in stage 3 is continued. If no immediate treatment given, the death occurs

- Pupillary asymmetry/dysfunction.
- Motor weakness.

The signs and symptoms of increased intracranial pressure in patient may depend on

1. The location of the lesion whether it is supratentorial or infratentorial.
2. The specific location of mass whether it is cerebral hemispheres, cerebellum or midbrain.
3. The degree of intracranial compensation.

Later findings

- Increased headache and vomiting
- Altered vital signs

- Respirator irregularities
- Continued deterioration in the level of consciousness
- Hemiplegia
- Decortication, decerebration, later, patient goes to deep coma which leads to death.

Investigation and Diagnosis

- History
- CT scan
- Blood investigation to look for any infection.

Management

Common protocols used in management of increased intracranial pressure are:

1. Surgery—if there is a localized mass or hematoma which can be removed by opening cranium or doing burrole.
2. Drug therapy to decrease the edema (like osmotic diuretics—e.g. mannitol, glycerine, steroids and anticonvulsants).
3. Fluid restriction
4. Hyperventilation
5. Temperature control
6. Cerebrospinal fluid drainage (Ventriculodrainage—cisternal puncture).

Nursing Management

The nurses' responsibility for the patient with acute increased intracranial pressure includes:

1. Provide continuous neurological assessment and maintain neurologic observation record. This can be done using a Glasgow coma scale in adults and Adelaide scale in children.
2. Maintenance of airway.
3. Prevention of activities that increase the intracranial pressure.
4. Fluid restriction.
5. Continuous intracranial pressure monitoring.
6. General nursing management.

1. Neurological Assessment

The Glasgow coma scale is now the most commonly used standardized assessment tool in the acute neurological environment worldwide. GCS enjoys a privileged position in the clinical and investigational context.

The GCS evaluates three types (Table 6.2) of behavior, i.e.

1. Eye opening
2. Verbal response
3. Motor response.

Response is elicited following the application of either a verbal or a painful stimuli. It is important to ensure that an adequate stimulus is applied otherwise a misleading response may be observed. The score can be applied which awards 1 point for the poorest response in all the three categories.

Table 6.2: Glasgow coma scale

Patient Name:	*Neuro No.*										*Ward:*
	Date and time										
Eyes open	Spontaneously 4										C=Eyes closed by swelling
	To command 3										
	To pain 2										
	No response 1										
Best motor response	Obeys commands 6										Record best arm response
	Localizes pain 5										
	Flexion-withdrawal 4										
	Flexion (abnormal) 3										
	Extension (abnormal) 2										
	No response 1										
Best verbal response	Oriented 5										T=Endotracheal tube or tracheostomy A=Aphasia
	Confused 4										
	Inappropriate words 3										
	Incomprehensible										
	Sounds 2										
	No response 1										
	Total score										

How to score responses on GCS (Glasgow coma scale) ?

Eye Opening

- Score 4 – Opens the eyes spontaneously
- Score 3 – Opens the eyes responding to calls
- Score 2 – Opens the eyes to painful stimuli
- Score 1 – Does not open the eyes even to painful stimuli

Motor Response

- Score 6 – Obeys simple commands
- Score 5 – Moves the limb to locate painful stimuli
- Score 4 – Attempts to withdraw the limb from source of pain
- Score 3 – Flexes arms and elbows in response to painful stimuli
- Score 2 – Extends arms to painful stimuli
- Score 1 – No motor response to painful stimuli

Verbal Response

- Score 5 – Oriented to time, place and person
- Score 4 – Able to converse things not oriented to time, place and person
- Score 3 – Can speak only words, not phrases or sentences
- Score 2 – Doing only incomprehensive sounds
- Score 1 – Does not respond verbally at all

Maximum Score is 15

Below 7 – It is explained the patient is in coma

Below 3 – It is explained as the patient is in deep coma.

Glasgow coma scale was used for both adults and children for few years. Later, a few great people in neuronursing thought of its inadequacy to be used for children because the children may not be able to respond verbally as it is shown in GCS. Yager *et al* investigated a number of the pediatric coma scales that have been devised to establish which was the most reliable. There were six scales designed and compared at different levels. Finally the Adelaide scale developed by Sampson and Reilly which is based on the proven formula of the Glasgow coma scale, found favour and is accepted superior to other formulae. The Adelaide scale incorporates changes to the verbal responses only to GCS. The eye and motor responses remain unaltered. Table 6.3 in the following page shown the differences between the adult and pediatric scales.

An important additional feature of the pediatric chart is the indication of the age-related norms for a particular age group. This is intended to guide staff in their observations and should only be used as an arbitrary guide.

Pediatric Coma Scale

Adelaide Scale

The Adelaide scale has been in clinical use since 1975. It is designed to assess conscious level in children under 5 years of age and is dependent on the idea that neurological immaturity needs to be considered when assessing children. This is taken into account by accepting that, in normal young subjects, the expected verbal and motor responses are lower than those in normal adults; this is in contrast to the adapted Pinderfield scale, in which children are not 'down-graded'.

Table 6.3: Comparison of Glasgow coma (adult) scale and Adelaide pediatric scale

Glasgow coma scale		*Adelaide pediatric coma scale*	
Response	*Score*		*Score*
Eyes open			
• Spontaneously	4		
• To speech	3		
• To pain	2	As adult scale	
• None	1		
Best verbal response			
• Oriented	5	• Oriented	5
• Confused	4	• Words	4
• Inappropriate words[1]	3	• Vocal sounds	3
• Incomprehensible sounds	2	• Cries	2
• None	1	• None	1
Best motor response			
• Obeys commands	5		
• Localizes to pain	4	As adult scale	
• Flexion to pain [2]	3		
• Extension to pain	2		
• None	—		

[1]The term 'monosyllabic response' may also be used.

[2]Flexion may be divided into abnormal and normal flexion, thus creating a 6-point scale.

Explanatory Notes on the Pediatric Coma Scale

Eyes Open

Spontaneously	If the patient's eyes open when first approached. Score 4 points.
To speech	If the eyes are not open at the start of the examination, speak to him, and if he opens his eyes. Score 3 points.
To pain	If verbal stimulation is unsuccessful, exert pressure on the patient's fingernail bed by a pencil, or pinch him gently. Score 2 points.
No response	Score 1 point.

Best Verbal Response

Orientated	After rousing the patient, ask him such questions as who and where he is. Children over five should be able to answer these; if correct, Score 5 points.
Words	The patient produces recognizable words, but is unable to give correct answers about orientation. This is normal from two to five years, but probably abnormal thereafter. Score 4 points.
Vocal sounds	The patient speaks or exclaims in a word or two, but without relevance to the examination. This may be normal in a young infant. Score 3 points.
Cries	The child cries or grunts, but does not achieve recognizable words; this is normal in the first twelve months. Score 2 points.
None	If no cry or grunt is produced, score 1 point.

Best Motor Response

Obeys orders	Ask the patient to "open your eyes" or "put out your tongue". Score 5 points.
Localise pain	If the patient does not obey commands, stimulate by pressure over the supraorbital notch—a positive response is an attempt to locate the painful stimulus and to remove it. Gentle pinching is also acceptable. Score 4 points.

Flexion response	After painful stimulus, the arm bends at the elbow but does not achieve a localizing response when stimulated at other sites. Score 3 points.
Extension response	In response to stimulation, the elbow straightens. Score 12 points.
None	If there is no motor response to strong painful stimulation. Score 1 point.

Total Scores

To be recorded by doctor or nurse

An older child, if conscious and alert, should score 14 points (E –4, V – 5, M – 5).

A younger child might be expected to score less, e.g. 12 (E – 4, V – 4, M – 4).

Neurological Observation in Children under 5 Years of Age

Verbal Response

In a baby under 6 months of age, the best verbal response is a cry, though it is recognized that some babies do make some vocal responses like 'ma', 'ba'. That means the expected best score for the child is 2 rather than 5. A child over 12 months of age will vocalize certain basic words like mummy, daddy.

A child above 5 years of age is expected to have the orientation to place and person, if not for time.

Motor responses are also assessed taking into account the expected neurological maturity for a particular age group.

The best motor responses that can be expected in a baby of 6 months is flexion. This is when the arm bends at the elbow following application of a painful stimulous to the fingernail bed.

In a children 6 months to 2 years of age localization would be expected.

Localization is recorded when the patient moves a limb in a particular way, to locate a painful stimuli. The stimulus is usually applied to the head and trunk. The trapezius pinch appears to be gaining popularity over supraorbital pressure, as it is easier and safer. The trapezius pinch is performed by pinching the trapezius muscle of the shoulder. Stimulation to supraorbital ridge is by resting the hand on the patients' forehead and placing the flat of the thumb on the supraorbital ridge, and applying a pressure.

Obeying commands—Child over 2 years of age should be able to obey simple commands. Extension is an abnormal finding. It is the straightening of the elbow in response to a painful stimulus. It may be accompanied by inward rotation of the shoulder and forearm with the wrist flexed and fingers straightened.

This is the details of the way the neurological observation is done in adult and children clinically. Along with GCS or Adelaide scale, vital signs chart and pupillary reaction chart are to be recorded.

Maintenance of Airway

Before doing anything to a critical patient anywhere in the medical field is to keep the airway clear and clean. This is applicable in neuroclinical set up also. The nurse can do the clearing and keeping the airway patent by:

- Keeping an appropriate airway if needed to prevent the tongue from back fall.
- Keeping the patient in lateral position if no contraindication.
- Do suctioning whenever is necessary.
- Intubate the patient if necessary.
- Use artificial ventilators if needed.

Prevention of Activities which can Increase the Intracranial Pressure

The nurse can prevent the increase of intracranial pressure by:

- Low suctioning while clearning the airway.
- Fluid restriction.
- Administration of antiedemic drugs.
- Preventing constipation which causes strain on defecation and in turn increases the pressure on the cranialcavity.
- Frequent, unnecessary shift of patient from bed to stretcher or stretcher to bed—this can be prevented by using wheeled beds.
- Keeping the environment free from dust which can prevent sneezing and coughing.
- Avoid elevation of body temperature.

Fluid Restriction

The nurse has to restrict the fluid intake of the patient by:

- Strict intake and output chart.
- Observing any change in the conscious level of patient and regulate the fluid accordingly.

Continuous Cranial Pressure Monitoring

This is done by the nurse, using
- Pressure monitors if possible by using ventilators where the intracranial pressure can be monitored.
- If above said instruments are not available, use of Glasgow coma scale is advisable.

General Nursing Management

This is done by the nurse by: (i) preventing
- Pressure sores
- Systemic infections
- Local infection
- Bladder and bowel dysfunction
- Footdrop
- Contractures, and (ii) taking care of early ambulation and enhancing early rehabilitation.

This chapter discusses the most important and vital responsibilities of a nurse in neurological and neurusurgical nursing.

APHASIA PATIENTS

Definition

The inability to communicate verbally is called aphasia. It can otherwise be defined as an acquired disorder of communication affecting the ability to comprehend and produce language. This formal definition means that the client, following some kind of brain damage has lost the ability to ask and answer questions to give and follow directions, to share feelings and emotions.

Anatomy and Physiology of Speech

One of the large area of cerebral function is communication. The motor speech area is located in the frontal lobe, anterior to laryngeal area in the premotor region of motor cortex, which is known as 'Brocas area'. In right-handed persons, the area is more developed in the left hemisphere and in the left handed persons, in the right hemisphere. The basis of language is a series of memory, pictures. The mind must know and recall the names of things in order to mention them. It must have seen or heard things in order to describe them and to have learned the words to express them. Even this is not enough. All these factors must work together under the influence of the center for articulate speech, which is in close connection with the larynx, tongue, and the muscles of the face.

Any injury to these centers results in some form of inability to speak, write, and to understand the written or spoken words. According to those inabilities, the aphasia can be mainly classified into two:

1. Motor aphasia/expressive aphasia
2. Sensory aphasia/receptive aphasia.

These can be further divided into:

1. Auditory receptive aphasia—lesion is in Wernick's area of the temporal lobe.
2. Visual receptive aphasia (Alexia)—lesion in parietal occipital area.
3. Expressive speaking aphasia—lesion in 'Brocas area' of frontal lobe.
4. Expressive writing aphasia (agraphia)—lesion at posterior frontal area.
5. Global aphasia—'involves both receptive and expressive aphasia'—lesions of Brocas area, Wernicks's area, Parietal area, occipital area, and posteral frontal area.

The aphasia can also be viewed in different levels in terms of impairment, the disability and the handicap.

The impairment is a disruption or a loss of, or a change in physiological structure or function. The impairment is identified by the name of the disease state. For example, 'hemorrhage', 'blood clot', 'vision loss' or 'hypertension'.

The goal of treatment for an impairment is prevention of further impairment.

The disability usually accompanies the symptoms of damage to the brain. This can be disability to think of a names, disability to follow directions, inability to read printed words, or inability to write cheques and so on. Here, the goal is to enhance the functional capacities and make the individual to compensate for impaired or lost skills and to maximize the use of residual skills.

The handicap of the aphasic patient is that the individual with brain damage experiences as a result of the impairment and disability. Here, the goal will be to educate others on patient's environment as well as the person with aphasia.

Assessment

1. History
   - Present
   - Past
2. Discourse sample
   - Conversational interview
   - Probe questions
   - Picture description
   - Stimulus question
3. Auditory comprehension
4. Visual/reading comprehension
5. Oral expression
6. Written expression.

Treatment/Management

It is done according to the cause of aphasia and also according to the level of aphasia.

The Nursing Management

As speech pathology and the speech therapy are developed and established well, the nurses' responsibility is mainly focused on supportive measures. Nurse is actively involved in the treatment in inpatient settings along with neurophysicians and neurosurgeons. Later, she can be confined to the supportive strategies like

1. Crisis management—in acute stage as well as when the patient is at home.
2. Different strategies to alleviate depressive mood. It can be preventive or curative.
3. Educate the patient and others to alter the environment so that the communication is easier. This is done according to the detail evaluation and recording to the patient's abilities and disabilities.
4. Assist the patient and family to get the financial support for setting new environment and acquiring appliances if needed.

As the individual is different, his/her potential is different, availability of financial and social support is different. The program should be individually tailored. And also it may vary from time-to-time. So the program and support strategies also should be renewed periodically.

Nursing Interventions in the Inpatient Settings

A. *Improving communication by*
- Encouraging the patient to listen patiently.
- Giving the patient plenty of time to speak.
- Avoiding talking too fast or too loud.
- Using short sentences.
- Being consistent by using the same words to express same ideas.
- Providing visual clues.
- Keeping paper and pen to express if needed.
- Encouraging to use any type of gestures if needed.
- Reinforcing each correct response.
- Using as many sensory channels as possible to stimulate the speech.

B. *Enhancing self concept by*
- Giving the patient as much as psychological security and support.
- Treating the patient as an individual normal adult.
- Avoiding forcing speech.
- Giving him/her chance to be in the social group to increase the self concept.
- Being patient to listen the patient.

C. *Crisis nursing intervention management*
- Accept him/her as an individual.
- Give him enough time to speak/express.
- Encourage him/her to use gestures to express.
- Use different gestures and sensory channels to stimulate the speech.
- Keep paper and pen to use in case of inability to express.
- Give alarm bells to use in case of emergency.
- Use short sentences while communicating.
- Treat him/her as a normal intellectual adult.
- Avoid forcing speech.
- Give eye to eye contact while conversing.

D. *Alleviate depressive mood*
- Encourage to come to social gathering if possible.
- Give opportunity to talk to the people who have recovered from aphasia.
- Use antidepressant if needed.
- Reading can be encouraged if needed to engage him/her.
- Encourage any other hobbies to spend the time.

E. *Alteration of the environment for effective communication*
- Use gestures and signs while talking.
- Educate the family members to accept him and be supportive.
- Encourage him to involve in the group.
- Do not isolate him in a separate room but keep him in a place where other family members interact with each other.
- Books with pictures of common articles used in daily life can be given which can be used for communication.
- Positive reinforcement to be given for good efforts of communication.

F. *Promoting the family coping*
- Explain the prognosis of the condition.
- Ask them to accept the patient as he is.
- Help them to change the environment to stimulate the speech like TV, VCR, transistor.
- Help them to change the environment to facilitate easy communication by giving calling bells to patient, pen and pad to write and communicate.
- Advice them to use all efficient communication methods with gestures, pictures, etc.
- Help them to get assistance if needed for appliance like hearing aid, etc.

7

Urinary Incontinence—Management

Urinary incontinence is a health problem of all ages and both sexes. A large number of people admitted to hospitals may have urinary incontinence temporary or permanently.

Incidence

Some studies show that 90 percent of human being experience urinary incontinence at least once in lifetime. Other studies tells that prevalence of urinary incontinence is estimated at 10 to 15 percent in the community based elderly and 50 to 60 percent in the institutionalized elderly. The prevalence is at a ratio of 9.5 in females and 2.2 percent in males. This problem adds the additional physical problems like, skin breakdown, falls, urinary tract infections, psychological problems like personal embarrassment, shame, guilt, dependency. So it is a problem which attracts a great attention of nursing population.

Definition

International continence society defined urinary incontinence as a condition in which involuntary loss of urine is 'a social or hygienic problem and is objectively demonstrated'. Thomas *et al* defined the incontinence as the involuntary excretion or leakage of urine in inappropriate places or at inappropriate times twice or more than a month, regardless of the quantity of urine loss.

Physiology of Urinary System

BRAIN →PONS → CONTROL STORAGE
+ EVACUATION
PARASYMPATHETIC SYSTEM → DETRUSOR TO CONTRACT
+ EMPTY THE BLADDER

REVIEW OF ANATOMY AND PHYSIOLOGY OF URINARY TRACT

Diagrammatic presentation of urinary tract

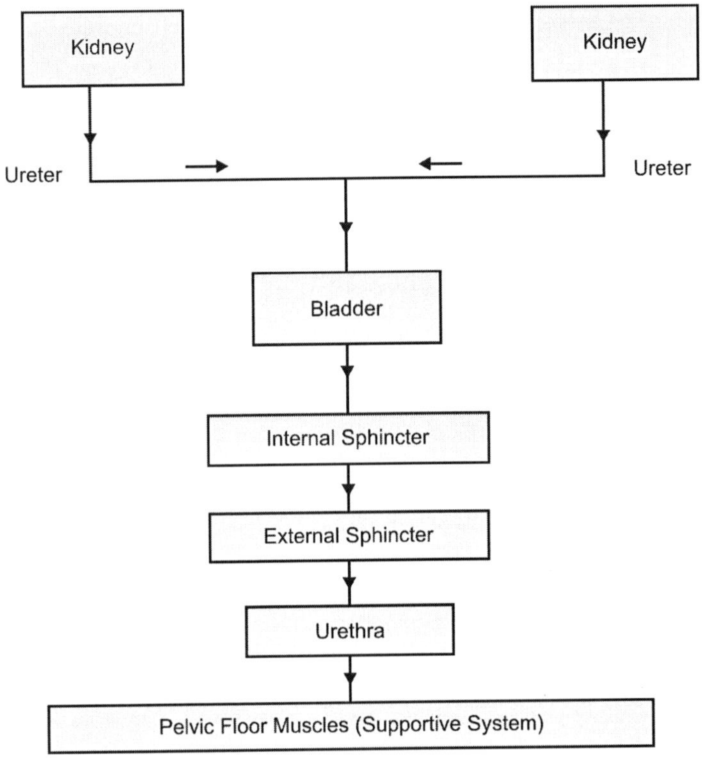

SYMPATHETIC NERVOUS SYSTEM → INTERNAL SPHINCTER TO CONTRACT

PUDENTAL NERVE → PELVIC FLOOR MUSCLES TO CONTRACT + THE EXTERNAL SPHINCTER

Normal micturation path is divided into:

Filling Phase

Where the detrusor muscles contract and the bladder fills with urine where the internal and external sphincter also contract to hold the urine in the bladder with the help of pelvic floor muscular tone.

Emptying Phase

Detrusor relax, internal and external sphincter also relax, urethra opens and urine is evacuated.

Causes of Urinary Incontinence

Anatomical causes

a. Any obstruction anywhere in urinary tract, e.g. presence of stones.
b. Any congenital abnormalities in urinary system, e.g. small bladder.
c. Any obstruction anywhere in urinary tract caused by the structural changes in the adjacent organs, e.g. pregnancy, tumor in uterus, constipation, enlarged prostate, etc.
d. Any anatomical change due to repeated childbirth, instrumental deliveries, hormonal changes in female, e.g. VVF, RVF, prolapse of uterus, menopause.
e. Injuries to brain, spinal cord T4 to S4, tumors of brain or spinal cord.

Hormonal causes

a. Diabetes.
b. Craniopharyngioma.

Types of Urinary Incontinence (Table 7.1)

1. *Urge incontinence:* This is the involuntary loss of urine associated with a strong desire to void.
2. *Stress incontinence:* It is involuntary loss of urine associated with increased intra-abdominal pressure, e.g. coughing, sneezing, lifting of heavy weight, etc.
3. *Overflow incontinence:* This is an involuntary loss of urine associated with over distention of the bladder. This type of incontinence may have variety of presentation, including frequent or constant dribbling, or stress incontinence symptoms.
4. *Functional incontinence:* Urine loss, may be associated with factors outside the lower urinary tract such as chronic impairment of physical or cognitive functioning or both.
5. *Transient incontinence:* It is only rare and for short period. It can occur in
   - Delirium
   - Infection of urinary tract

- Atrophic vaginitis
- Pharmaceutical
- Psychological
- Endocrine disorder
- Restricted mobility
- Stool impaction.

METHODS OF INVESTIGATION OR EVALUATION AND DIAGNOSIS

Evaluation and diagnosis can be done under the following headings:

1. History
   a. Urogynecological
   b. Menstrual
   c. Gynecological
   d. Obstetric
   e. Surgical
   f. Medical
2. Physical examination
   a. General
   b. Systemic
3. Laboratory tests
   Urine analysis
   a. Routine
   b. Culture and sensitivity
4. Urodynamics
   a. Residual urine volume
   b. Filling cystometry
   c. Voiding cystometry
   d. Urethral pressure outflowmetry
   e. Video cystourethrography
   f. Ambulatory urodynamics
5. Other simple tests
   a. Pad test,
   b. Incontinence chart,
   c. Residual urine
6. Others
   a. Screening cystourethrography
   b. Vaginal ultrasound
   c. Cystourethroscopy
   d. Intravenous urethrography.

Table 7.1: Types, causes and pathology of urinary incontinence

Types	*Causes*	*Pathology*
Stress incontinence	Weakness of pelvic floor Bladder outlet weakness	Reduced outlet resistance
Urge incontinence	Detrusor motor and/or sensory instability, isolated or associated with local genitourinary condition – such as cystitis, urethritis, tumors, stones or outflow obstruction CNS disorder such as stroke, dementia, parkinsonism, spinal cord injury or disease, anatomic obstruction by prostate structure, cystocele	Overactive detrusor
Retention overflow	A contractile bladder associated with diabetes mellitus Or spinal cord injury, obstruction from detrusor, sphincter dyssynergia	Increased outlet resistance and underactive detrusor
Functional	Severe dementia and other neurological disorders Psychological factors such as depression, regression, anger and hostility	Severe physical and mental disabilities, unconductive environment that cannot be modified

Management

Management is varying according to the cause of the urinary incontinence. Management can be medical, surgical or environmental manipulation.

As the handbook is for the use of nursing population, the nursing management will be discussed in the following pages.

Nursing Management: Three Objectives

1. For the independent continence
2. For the dependent continence
3. For the social continence.

Independent continence: It means the patient himself/herself is able to control his incontinence and become fully continent.

Dependent continence: Here the patient depends upon other people to become continent—e.g. using intermittent catheterization or continous catheterization getting help to get into the toilet, strip the clothing before urinating.

Social continence: Here the patient uses some measures to make him/her continent when he/she in a group of people, so that he need not be withdrawn from the society or working place—e.g. using absorbent, pads, using clip to the penis, urine pouches, etc.

Assessment

During assessment by nurses, the assessment tool given below can be used:

Incontinence Assessment Tool

Name: Age: Sex:

Medication currently taking 1.
2.
3.

Duration of the medication

Date of onset of incontinence________________

Precipitating factor – emotional upset – exhaustion,

Frequency - day/night/both

Do you get wet when:
- Coughing
- Sneezing
- Standing
- Turning over in bed
- Delayed to reach bathroom
- When excited
- Leaving bathroom.

When you urinate, does it:
- Burn
- Itch
- Stink
- Foul smell
- Look cloudy
- Dribble

When you urinate is it:
- Small amount
- Large amount
- Dribble

Do you have difficulty in:
- Walking to bathroom
- Getting into commode
- Getting clothes up/down

Is the incontinence related:
- To constipation
- Increased fluid consumption

Can you:
- Stop urinating at will
- Start urinating at will
- Wait to get a commode
- Feel the urge to urinate
- Sense when voiding occurs

Do you:
- Stay home because of incontinence
- Wear pads or use other aids

- Soil clothing or furniture
- Feel anxious or embarrassed

Is your condition:

- Unchanged
- Improved
- More severe

Do you get relieved with any measures if you have taken:

This assessment tool gives you a guideline what will be the cause and type of incontinence roughly.

Nursing Measures/Strategies for the Management of Urinary Incontinence

They can be listed as follows:

a. Deal with constipation
b. Deal with urinary tract infection
c. Behavioral techniques
d. Pelvic floor exercises
e. Intermittent catheterization
f. Indwelling catheterization
g. Provide aids like—external male collection system
    - Pouches
    - Absorbent pads

    The main aim of the nursing management should be
    - to restore the continence and
    - to prevent the deterioration of the upper urinary tract.

8

Pain—Management

Pain is a complex phenomena. The understanding of pain has undergone and still undergoing changes. Pain in different systems of the human body gives different experience to the individual. Pain experienced with a sharp instrument is different from a colicky pain of the alimentary system. Pain due to an insect bite is different from a pain due to an infection in the throat. Pain from blunt injuries are different from a stab injury. So pain can have very many varying expressions in different situations.

People from different countries and different branches of medicine and paramedicals tried to define pain. But no definition is agreed upon unanimously. A purely physiological definition can be "pain is a protective mechanism". Malzack and Wall (1988) describe pain as a complex experience encompassing sensory, emotional, cognitive and behavioural components. International Association for the Study of Pain (IASP) defines pain as the sensation caused by noxious (i.e. tissue damaging) or potentially tissue damaging stimuli (1986). For the nurse an appropriate definition is, pain is what the patient says it is, existing when he says it does (Mc Caffery 1983). Each definition is not complete in itself though it gives some views of pain, so more comprehensive definition of pain can be expected in coming years.

Components of Pain

1. Sensory discriminative—is recognition of the sensation of pain.
2. Affective motivational component—is the emotional and behavioral dimension of pain.
3. Cognitive—is the evaluative component in the responses to the pain experience that are determined by past experience, learned behaviors, etc. When one looks at the components of pain, one can understand that many factors influence the individual in

experiencing and expressing the pain. When a person has normal sensory pathways, if the emotional behavior of the individual is well-controlled, the expression of the pain may be less severe. And also the person who experiences pain repeatedly also can tolerate the pain better, where the expression of pain may not be that severe. The common factors influencing the expression of pain are :

- Gender (sex)
- Past experience
- Age
- Personality—emotional control
- Body part affected
- Meaning of pain to that individual in that situation.

The Mechanism of Pain

Pain stimuli: Tissue damage can be caused by physical or chemical stimuli. Or it can be from a mechanical, heat or chemical source.

These stimuli also can be endogenous or exogenous. Exogenous can be acid, bases, heat, and so on. Endogenous may be potassium, histamine, serotinin, acetylcholine, etc.

Nociceptors: Pain receptors are called nociceptors. Some receptors respond to only one type of pain stimuli. Others respond to any noxious stimuli and for nonpain producing stimuli like pressure stimuli.

Pain pathways: Pain stimuli, responded by nociceptors travel towards the spinal cord through an afferent nerve fiber, from the anterolateral system of the spinal cord it reaches brainstem. Brainstem areas have numerous connections with hypothalamus and limbic system. This results in increased sympathetic tone, tachycardia, increased cardiac output and hypertension. The activation of limbic system also caused the emotional responses to the pain experienced in the individual.

Pain perception: Pain perception probably takes place at thalamic level from thalamic region the impulses reach the cortex. The cortex is presumed to provide analysis and interpretation of pain experience. The interpretation of the type, quality and meaning of pain is influenced by different factors like cultural background, motivation in life, personality, age, sex, etc. It also has descending pathways acts at three levels—at the midbrain level opiates are released. This also activates a system of serotinin—containing cells at medullary level. This system transmits inhibitory impulses to the cells in the dorsal horn. Serotinin plays an important role in the function of the descending pain system.

Schematic Representation of Pain Mechanism

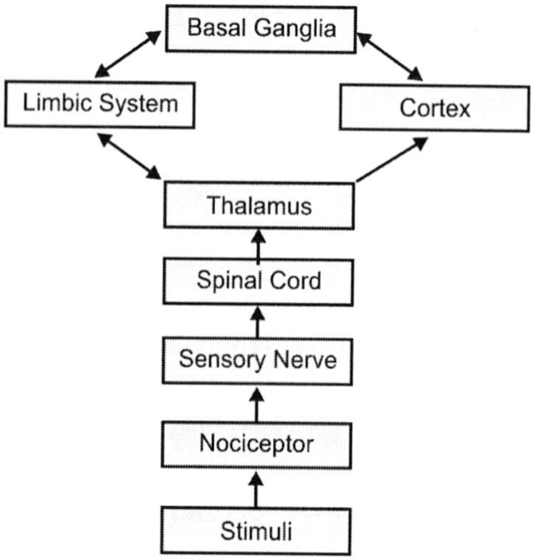

Neurotransmitters are involved in pain mechanism. Among the neurotransmitters, neuropeptide such as encephaline and endorphins play an important role in inhibiting pain.

As a whole pain transmission is a complex process involving peripheral and central mechanisms that interact dynamically to receive, monitor and modulate the pain experience. Whether the stimuli are perceived as painful or not, depends on a variety of factors which interplay with the central mechanisms at the cortex and the limbic system.

Based upon the researches done to understand the mechanism of pain, a few theories are formed and published. The major pain theories are:

1. The specificity theory
2. The pattern theory
3. The thalamic neuron theory
4. The gate control theory.

1. *The specific theory* was proposed by Deseartes in 17th century. This is the earliest theory regarding pain. This theory talks about the special receptors which are responsible for pain. This theory does not explain about the pain tolerance. It give explanation for ablative neurosurgical procedures.
2. *The pattern theory* does not talk much about the special receptors of pain. This theory tells that pain is experienced because various sensory receptors are stimulated in a definite pattern. The pattern theory contributed many factors in the understanding of pain, but very little about the influence of psychological factors in the perception of pain.
3. *The thalamic neuron theory* suggests that thalamic neurons are responsible for chronic pain. This theory brings pain generation from periphery to the thalamus.
4. *The gate control theory* was proposed in 1965 but explained in 1967 and 1976. According to this theory, pain results from a balance of input to central transmission through myelinated and unmyelinated fibers. This theory is more useful in clinical practice.

Types of Pain Syndrome

Acute Pain

It is explained as a sudden unpleasant sensory, emotional experience caused by accidental injury, with sharp instruments, insect bites, fall, blunt injuries, burn, surgical procedures, etc. If the causative factors are not removed or the cycle is not broken by effective management it becomes gradually chronic.

Chronic Pain

Chronic pain is referred to as a pain which occurs recurrently and extends over a period of 6 months. It can be due to post-traumatic, postinfections, vascular, degenerative or idiopathic. Postoperative pain and post-traumatic pain are other forms of pain syndromes which are self-explanatory.

The gate control theory and the inhibiting mechanism of endogenous opiates give support for the clinical practice of rubbing, massaging, touch, acupuncture and electrical stimulation.

Above said pain theories talk about different aspects of pain and some are useful in clinical practice.

Age Related Pain Tolerance

It is contradictory that whether the aging can increase or decrease the pain tolerance. Generally people believe that aging increases the pain tolerance. The reasons may be:

- Decreased number of active peripheral nerves
- Decreased number of pain receptors
- Drug therapy for any other disease conditions
- Cognitive impairment
- Transmission of impulse may take increased time—so the perception is also delayed. But as a whole the age related reduction in pain is unexplained.

Assessment of Pain

Assessment of pain can be done by the followings:

1. Location of pain
2. Mode of onset (acute or chronic)
3. Any precipitating factors
4. Quality of pain (dull, moderate, shooting, spasms)
5. Duration
6. Any change in quality
7. Any measures taken after pain started, if so
   a. What measures
   b. Whether it is effective
8. Clinical observation
   a. Clients appearance
   b. Motor behavior (facial expression, gait, posture)
   c. Affective behavior
   d. Local 'Observation' if pain is external
9. Monitoring of vital and signs like BP, pulse, temperature.

Management of Pain

Techniques used for management of pain

Few techniques are used to produce analgesia in the individuals. These analgia is achieved through dermal stimulation using some techniques. The common techniques used in the skin are :

1. Pressure—Pressure applied by finger tips or thumb
2. Acupressure—It involves pressure and massage
3. Massage—Rubbing on and around the area of pain
4. Cutaneous vibration—Short and long wave diathermy

5. Heat therapy—Either dry heat or moist heat application
6. Cold therapy—Dry cold or moist cold application
7. External application—of gel or creams
8. TENS (transcutaneous electrical nerve stimulation—using electrical current through electrodes applied to the skin surface of the painful region).

The mechanism involved in all above said techniques is according to pain theories available. Some of these techniques produce exogenous opiates to control the pain. Others block the endogenous pain inducing substances. There are few deep structure. Therapies used in pain management are;

Acupuncture: It is a procedure, where needles are inserted at specific cutaneous sites. The effect is not immediate but opiates will be produced to control the pain.

Deep brain stimulation: Here electrical stimulation is done to the certain areas of brain including frontal lobes, midbrain, caudate nucleus etc.

Drugs used in Pain Management

1. *Analgesics:* May interfere with the pain transmission from periphery to center (cortex or thalamine). Some drugs alter the perception and response to pain.
2. *Narcotic analgesics:* These drugs alter the perception of pain experience and behavioral response to the pain.
3. *Nonsteroidal anti-inflammatory drug:* May usually act at the periphery inhibiting the transmitting substance which cause pain.
4. *Serotinine blockers:* They act on serotinine by blocking its receptors. Thus analgesia is produced.
5. *Anesthesia:* The functional part of the nervous system is temporarily or permanently destroyed to interrupt pain transmission from periphery to the spinal cord and cerebral cortex or thalamus.
6. *Nerve blocks:* For this local anesthetics are used. The effect may be for few hours. Usually used before any short surgical procedures.

Nursing Management of Pain

Pain is considered as a complex phenomena to understand and to assess as well. Pain has different components such as sensory, affective and cognitive. Each person has different biological and psychological factors which can effect the components of pain they have. So the assessment and management of pain also is difficult. Different people have written volumes for pain management. Carlliet is the author of 8 such books, namely:

- *Knee Pain and Disability*
- *Low Back Pain Syndromes*
- *Shoulder Pain*
- *Hand Pain and Impairment*
- *Neck Pain and Arm Pain*
- *Soft Tissue Pain and Disability*
- *Foot and Ankle Pain and Disability*
- *Head and Face Pain Syndrome.*

It shows the management of pain in different parts of the body is understood and evaluated differently and managed differently. It means the nursing management of different pain to be different, so it is difficult to note down the nursing management of each pain condition.

But in general nurse should be able to

- accept the patient as he is.
- accept and acknowledge the pain as what the patient feels or expresses.
- assist the individual to identify the situation when or where the pain started.
- assist the individual to identify the situation which intensify the pain.
- do the assessment using the performa available.
- assist/apply the prescribed pain management strategies like:
    i. Pressure
    ii. Massage
    iii. Heat therapy
    iv. Cold therapy
    v. Acupressure
    vi. Giving comfortable positions
    vii. TENS
- administer the drugs accordingly.
- give the individual to ventilate the feelings.
- give emotional support.
- give altered lifestyle to prevent situations which trigger the pain.

- family members can be involved in sessions.
- family members can be kept aware of the situation which can avoid the triggering of pain.
- family members can be taught some physical measures which can comfort the patient.

Most important nursing measure is to have a very good personal relationship to keep the patient physically and psychologically supported.

Pain and its management is undergoing changes still. So the nurses need to update their knowledge by reading the books/ articles, attending ongoing in-service programs or consulting the experts and peer groups for better pain management.

9

Infections of Nervous System

The nervous system and its covering can be infected by the same bacteria and viruses which affect other organs of the body and the illness so caused may be acute as in the case of poliomyelitis, subacute (some forms of encephalitis) or chronic as in neurosyphilis.

Inflammation of meninges is called meningitis, that of the brain encephalitis and the spinal cord myelitis. Neuritis means inflammation of peripheral nerve and polyneuritis means, the infection of many nerves. When the nerve root is affected the term radiculitis is used.

Infection may be caused by:

1. *Bacteria*
   a. Pyogenic organism: *Staphylococcus aureus*, pneumococci, meningococci.
   b. Nonpyogenic organism:

Tubercle bacilli	—	Neurotuberculosis
Spirochaeta	—	Neurosyphilis
Salmonella	—	Enteric fever

2. *Viruses*
   a. Japanese encephalitis
   b. Echoviruses
   c. Chickenpox, mumps, measles
   d. Herpes simplex
   e. Polio and nonpolio enteroviruses
   f. Rabies
3. *Fungi*
   a. *Cryptococcus*
   b. *Candida albicans*
4. *Parasites*
   a. Malarial parasite

b. Cysticercal cysts
c. Toxoplasma fungi
d. Trypanosomes.

Routes of Entry

The routes of entry of infection include the bloodstream, direct extension from the primary site, cerebrospinal fluid (CSF), extension along cranial and peripheral nerves, the mouth and nasopharynx and transmission *in utero.*

Bloodstream

This is the most common route by which the infectious microorganisms reach the CNS. Microorganism may enter the bloodstream as a result of insect bite, or spread of infection from primary foci. (Middle ear infection, mastoidities, sinusitis, cellulites or any other infections of the body).

Direct Extension from a Primary Site

Fracture of the frontal or facial bones, or any compound cranial fractures that create communication between the sterile intracranial area and the outside environment. This is a prime source for infection.

Cerebrospinal Fluid

Dural tear as a result of injury can create a connection between the CSF and the ear or nose. In otorrhea and rhinorrhea the microorganisms directly extend to CSF and infection develops. Poor sterile technique during lumbar puncture or spinal surgery can also contaminate CSF.

Extension along Cranial and Spinal Nerves

Some microorganisms reach the CNS by following the peripheral nerves, e.g. rabies.

Mouth and Nasopharynx

Some organisms are transmitted by oral and nasopharyngeal secretions, especially when people are in close contact, e.g. meningococcal meningitis.

In utero

The fetus *in utero* may also get CNS infection. The causes may be contaminated amniotic fluid from amniocentesis, any maternal infection, viruses such as rubella, etc.

MENINGITIS

Meningitis is an infection of the meninges. (The coverings of the brain and spinal cord). The infection is of any of the three layers, pia mater, arachnoid mater or dura mater. The subarachnoid space and the CSF are also usually involved.

There are three main types of meningitis:

a. Bacterial or pyogenic, i.e. caused by pus forming bacteria, the most common being meningococci, pneumococci and *H. influenzae* bacillus.
b. Tuberculosis caused by the tubercle bacilli.
c. Viral caused by a number of different viruses.

Bacterial Meningitis

Definition

Bacterial meningitis is a pyogenic (purulent) infection that involves the pia-arachnoid layers of the meninges and the subarachnoid space including CSF.

Causes

Pneumococci, meningococci, streptococci, staphylococci.

The most common causes of bacterial meningitis depends on the age of the patient.

- In newborn: *Streptococcus agalactiae*, gram-negative bacilli and *Listeria monocytogenes*
- In children: *Haemophilus influenzae, Neisseria meningitidis*, streptococcus
- Adults: *Streptococcus pneumoniae.*

Pathophysiology

When the bacteria invade the pia-arachnoid and subarachnoid spaces, initially blood supply to that area increases rapidly. Neutrophils soon migrate into the space and engulf the bacteria.

The phagocytic cells rapidly degenerate and disintegrate and form a purulent material within the subarachnoid space. The exudates increases and may even extend to perivascular space causing encephalitis. The veins become dilated and congested. If the inflammation extends through the walls of the veins (vasculitis), thrombosis or necrosis occurs. The irritation from bacteria and toxins causes swelling and an increase in endothelial cells. Neutrophils and lymphocytes migrate between the layers of the vessel with resulting fibrotic changes. Adhesions and effusions can develop in the subarachnoid space, thereby interfering with normal circulation of CSF. This may contribute to the development of hydrocephalus. Some organisms may produce abscesses. The outcome of bacterial meningitis depends on early and aggressive treatment to prevent development of complications.

Signs and Symptoms

The common symptoms of meningitis in young children include

- fever,
- anorexia,
- vomiting, diarrhea,
- listlessness,
- a shrill cry and bulging of fontanels.

In older adults Headache, vomiting, fever, detoriation in the level of consciousness (LOC), signs of meningeal irritations, general convulsions, increased ICP, cranial nerve dysfunction, endocrine disorders, others, (hypersensitivity, hyperalgesia, muscle hypotonia).

1. *Headache and fever:* Patient may have few days of pyrexia, a vague influenza like state, with cold and sore throat, later develop headache which is severe in nature, temperature may vary from 101 to 103 degrees. It may increase to 105 at the terminal stages, because of the decompression of increased ICP on the brainstem.
2. *Changes in level of consciousness:* It starts with shortened attention span and misinterpretation to stimuli and this leads to disorientation to time, place and person. Later patient may become drowsy, lethargic, and unresponsive may lapse into deep coma.
3. *Signs of meningeal irritation:*
   a. Stiff neck or neck rigidity is an early sign of meningeal irritation. Forceful flexion produces severe pain. This is

demonstrated by attempting unsuccessfully to bend the head forwards so as to bring the chin on to the chest.

b. *Kernig's sign:* Kernig's sign is elicited by flexing the upper leg at the hip to a 90° angle and then attempting to extend the knee. If meningitis is present, there is pain and spasm of the hamstrings when an attempt is made to extend the knee. The pain is due to the inflammation of the meninges and spinal root.
c. *Brudzinski's sign:* This sign is positive when both the upper leg at the hip and the lower leg at the knee flex in response to passive flexion of the neck and head on the chest. This reflex is caused by irritating exudates around the roots in the lumbar region.

4. *Generalised convulsions:* Development of generalized seizures indicates irritation of the cerebral cortex, transitory paralysis may be present after convulsions.
5. *Increase ICP:* Due to increase ICP vomitings are frequent. papilledema may be present.
6. *Endocrine disorders:* A small percentage of patients develop hyponatremia and excessive release of antidiuretic hormone. There will be signs and symptoms of water retentions. Limiting water intake is a part of management.
7. *Other signs:* Other symptoms noted include, skin hypersensitivity, hyperalgesia, and muscular hypotonia. If vascular supply to brain is affected, there may be hemiparesis dementia and aphasia.

Diagnosis

It is based on:

a. History and physical examination along with laboratory data. While taking history recent infections such as infections of ear, sinusus, respiratory track has to be traced out.
b. The organism is identified on the basis of CSF culture and Gram stain.

Management

Selection of antibiotics depends on age and risk factors. The treatment is directed at:

1. General supportive measures.

2. Antibacterial drug therapy.
3. Recognition and management of complications.

Supportive measures include maintenance of adequate ventilation and patent airway, maintaining fluid, and electrolyte balance, controlling high temperature, managing and controlling of seizures and headache.

Antibacterial therapy: Most adults are treated with ampicillin 200 mg/kg per day IV and ceftriaxine 200 mg/kg per day.

Injection dexamethasone 10 mg IV every 6th hourly for 4 days may be given in severe cases to reduce the severity of residual neurologic and cranial nerve damage.

Complications

Complications of bacterial meningitis depends on the type of causative organism and the severity of the illness. The post-meningitis sequele include.

- visual impairment,
- optic neuritis,
- deafness,
- personality change,
- headache,
- seizures,
- paresis, or paralysis,
- hydrocephalus,
- pneumonia,
- endocarditis,
- granulomas and abscesses.

Prevention

Bacterial meningitis can be prevented if the following principles are observed.

- Providing adequate treatment of infections such as sinusitis, mastoiditis, ear infection and pneumonias.
- Maintaining strict aseptic precaution during all intracranial and intraspinal operations and procedures.
- Maintaining aseptic technique in doing dressings of the procedure.
- Administering prophylactic antibiotics with skull fractures, dural tears and injuries causing CSF drainage from ear or nose.

Viral Meningitis (Aseptic Meningitis)

Viral meningitis is a self-limited illness seen most frequently in children and young adults. The presentation is similar to bacterial meningitis except that neurologic dysfunction (e.g. change in mental status, neurologic deficits) does not occur and the overall prognosis is good.

The diagnosis is suspected when CSF is found to be clear and contain mainly lymphocytes, while sugar and chlorides are normal and is confirmed by negative bacterial cultures. In some cases, the virus may be cultured from CSF, or from nasal, pharyngeal swabs. Treatment is symptomatic and supportive, no drug therapy is effective against the virus.

Chronic Meningitis: Tuberculous Meningitis

Tuberculous meningitis is caused by *Mycobacterium tuberculosis* which is a severe infection that carries a high morbidity and mortality.

The onset of this disease is much less acute. The patient may have been vaguely unwell for weeks with gradually increasing headache and listlessness. He may of course be known to have tuberculosis elsewhere. Evidence of active pulmonary disease is found in only 30 percent of cases and only 50 percent of the cases are purified protein derivative (PPD) positive. This is the common and treatable disease in India.

Signs and symptoms are like in the case of meningitis.

The clinical picture of tuberculosis meningitis is quite variable, with substantial differences among patients of different ages.

Staging system was introduced in 1947.

Stage I: Nonspecific manifestations of infection without neurologic symptoms and signs. No clouding of consciousness.

Stage II: Signs and symptoms of meningeal irritation with cranial nerve palsies but no other neurologic defects and no clouding of consciousness. Lethargy or alteration in behavior.

Stage III: Cross neurologic defect, stupor or coma

- Abnormal movement
- Convulsion
- Severe neurologic deficits (pareses).

In Children

- fever—constantly present
- nausea
- vomiting
- behavioral changes headache—25 percent of children and never identified patients under 3 year of age
- abdominal pain and constipation
- anorexia
- seizures—50 percent children and more frequent in younger children
- signs of meningeal irritation.

In Adults

Duration of symptoms generally 2 to 3 weeks before medical attention.

- Headache—(50 to 75%) is prominent complaint
- Nausea (less frequent)
- Behavioral changes—apathy—majority of patients confusion or bizarre behavior
- Fever (sign)
- Focal neurologic sign—unilateral or bilateral cranial nerve palsy.

Most frequently affected is sixth cranial nerve.

- Neurologic deficit—hemiparesis
- Fundus: Optic fundus may occasionally offer specific clues to the presence of TB meningitis
    i. visible tubercles in choroids
    ii. retinal lesions near optic disk
    iii. papilledema
- Hydrocephalus

  Diagnosis is done by CSF culture, X-ray chest, CT scan and MRI.

Treatment

Until antibiotic sensitivity is known, treatment with four drugs is recommended for the first 2 months. A full course of treatment requires 9 to 12 months. Options include

- Isoniazid 300 mg per day (also give pyridoxine 50 mg per day),
- Rifampin 600 mg per day,
- Pyrazinamide 15 to 30 mg/kg per day,

- Ethambutol 15 to 20 mg/kg per day, streptomycin 15 mg/kg per day IM, and
- Ciprofloxacin 750 mg two times a day.
- Cotreatment with dexamethasone 10 mg IV every 6 hours may also be used in severe cases (with depressed level of consciousness, focal deficits, or multiple cranial nerve palsies) to inhibit the inflammatory response and limit damage.

Surgical Treatment

Surgical intervention in tuberculosis meningitis is primarily directed at relief of hydrocephalus. Ventricular drainage may be done to relieve pressure.

ENCEPHALITIS

Inflammation of the brain is called encephalitis. If the meninges are involved at the same time it is called meningoencephalitis.

Causes

It is caused by viruses, bacteria, fungi or parasites. Viruses are the most common offending organism. Other less frequent causes of encephalitis include toxic substances, such as ingested lead or arsenic or inhaled carbon monoxide, vaccines for measles, mumps and rabies, which cause postvaccination encephalitis and viral infections such as measles, mumps, etc.

Signs and Symptoms

The symptoms depend upon the kind of organisms and the area affected. The basic syndrome of viral encephalitis is characterized by fever, headache, vomiting, confusion, seizure , stiffness of neck and change in level of consciousness, which varies from disorientation, agitation, restlessness, drowsiness and finally to coma. The patient may develop neurologic deficits such as aphasia or mutism, hemiparesis, ataxia, ocular paralysis, etc.

Treatment is antibiotics, supportive and symptomatic.

Nursing Management of Patients with Acute Meningitis/ Encephalitis/Chronic Meningitis

In the acute stage of meningitis, the patient appears to be seriously ill. The nursing management regardless of etiology is directed towards:

1. Assessment of patient condition
2. Providing supportive care
3. Adhering to specific protocol
4. Preventing complications and
5. Rehabilitation.

1. Assessment of Patient Condition

Patient should be assessed for vital conditions, like

- Level of consciousness,
- Pupillary reaction and
- Respiratory function.

2. Basic Supportive Care like

a. Maintain a patient airway
   - Patient should be kept on sidelying position
   - Suction to be done as and when necessary

b. Maintain adequate oxygenation
   - Administer oxygen therapy
   - Monitor blood gases
   - Assess frequently for signs and symptoms of dyspnea and cyanosis.

c. Administer basic hygienic care

d. Protect the patient from injury
   - Putting the cot's side rails up
   - Observing frequently

e. Control high temperature
   - Remove excess bed clothes
   - Give tepid bath if temperature is high
   - Administer antipyretic drugs
   - Maintain a cool room temperature
   - Use hypothermia blanket

f. Lessen headache
   - Elevate the head to 30 degrees
   - Apply an ice cap
   - Maintain a quiet darkened room
   - Administer analgesic if ordered

g. Provide adequate nutrition
   - Ryles tube feed, second hourly if the patient has altered level of consciousness
   - Fluid intake and output chart to be maintained

In adults, fluid intake to be maintained a level of 2500 ml in 24 hours.

- Supplementary vitamins to be given

h. Monitor blood investigations like blood sugar, electrolytes, renal and liver functions.

i. Provide emotional support to patient and family.

3. Specific Protocol

Patient with meningitis is hypersensitive to the environmental stimuli.

a. So provide a quiet environment in a darkroom where the patient is kept in strict bedrest, control environmental noise, control direct light.

b. Seizure activity common in patient with CNS infection, so maintain seizure precautions.

c. Observe for increased intracranial pressure and incorporate nursing protocol to manage the increased intracranial pressure.

4. Prevention of Complications

The duration of the acute and chronic phase of meningitis depends on many variables. However, specific nursing protocol is to be followed to prevent complications like

- skin breakdown,
- lung complications,
- thrombophlebitis and
- deformities.

Observe for signs of adrenal insufficiency in the patient with meningococcal meningitis like hypotension, respiratory collapse, petichiae, so that immediate interventions may be taken to preserve patient's life.

NEUROSYPHILIS

Neurosyphilis is an infection of any part of the nervous system resulting from infection by spirochaeta, *Treponema pallidum*. It develops after inadequate treatment of early syphilis.

Primary infection of syphilis is characterized by a chancre (firm painless genital ulcer).

A secondary bacteremic stage may occur 2 to 12 weeks later and this results in generalized mucocutaneous lesions (Palmar and Plantar rash) and lymphadenopathy. Two percent of patients with secondary infection experience acute meningovascular syphilis.

Following latent period of 15 to 20 years tertiary syphilis manifests as a slowly progressive systemic inflammatory diseases of the skin (gummas), heart (aortitis) and eyes (chorioretinitis).

Tertiary neurosyphilis develops in 7 percent of patients with untreated primary syphilis and results in chronic meningeal and parenchymal inflammation.

Pathology

Pathology is extensive and include the meninges, blood vessels, brain, spinal cord and peripheral nerves. The meninges are congested and the pia-arachnoid is infiltrated with lymphocytes that gather around blood vessels. The blood vessels show proliferation of the intima. Splitting of the elastica and cellular infiltration resulting severe panarteritis. Lack of blood supply due to arterial disease results in atrophy. This is most striking in the frontal lobes. The spinal cord shows degeneration of the posterior tracts and the peripheral nerves show loss of the large calibered sensory fibers.

Signs and Symptoms

This condition produces three main diseases. The classic manifestations include:

1. Meningovascular syphilis
2. Tabes dorsalis
3. General paralysis of the insane (GPI).

Meningovascular syphilis: The infection involves the meninges and blood vessels causing them to be inflamed and thickened. Blood vessel walls becomes narrowed. Episodes of thrombosis occur causing sudden paralysis of one of the cranial nerves or a limb.

CSF shows slightly raised lymphocyte count and the blood WR will usually be positives. Many parts of the nervous system can be involved.

Tabes dorsalis: The signs and symptoms of this disorder are mainly due to degeneration of the dorsal (posterior) part of the spinal cord (Tabes = Wasting).

Here the sensory roots are affected. Patient will have

- Lightning pains—they are sudden bursts of needle like pains that shins calves and arms.
- Girdle pains—prolonged sensations resembling a constriction band around the trunk.
- Loss of position sense—patient becomes ataxic and walks with legs wide apart with a stamping gait.
- Tendon reflex will be absent so no bladder control will be present.
- Ulcers on the feet due to loss of sensation.
- Gross destructive changes in the knees and other joints leads to disorganized joints charcot's joints. This will be painless due to loss of sensory fibers.
- Argyll Robertson pupil—This is a small irregular pupil which does not react to light but does constrict on looking at a near object. This is the most characteristic sign of neurosyphilis in the eyes.

General paralysis of the insane (GPI): In this type of neurosyphilis the nerve cells of the brain are involved. Many of them die and the brain atrophies or shrinks.

The Symptoms are:

- Slow mental deterioration leading to dementia.
- Prominent psychiatric features. Patient may have grandiose delusions, emotional changes.
- fits.

Diagnosis is done by:

- Blood investigations including VDRL.
- Lumbar puncture.

Treatment

- Primary and secondary syphilis can be treated with benzathine penicillin 24 million units IM weekly for 3 weeks.
- Neurosyphilis whether latent or active is treated with penicillin G2 to 4 million units IV every 4th hours for 10 days.

Nursing Care

It is difficult to discuss the nursing care of neurosyphilis patient as the patient presents diverse signs and symptoms with every degree of disability from slight ataxia to the complete dependence of a demented bedridden patient. So care should be individualized according to the patient's symptoms.

- Nurse should be aware that no barrier nursing precautions are necessary during the tertiary stage of the disease.
- All the patients with neurosyphilis should be encouraged to be as active and independent as possible.
- Epilepsy is a common symptom of meningovascular and general paralytic forms of neurosyphilis so seizure precautions should be provided in the care.
- Patients with delusions of grandeur should not be contradicted. Ways and means should be found to deter any unacceptable behavior. Sometimes tranquilizers may be given to calm the patient.
- The patient with tabes dorsalis should be taught to take particular care of his skin and painless ulcers of the feet. They should wear comfortable easy fitting shoes to prevent development of corns and abrasions on feet.
    a. Charcoats joints—patients should be taught to walk as correctly as possible using walking aids.
    b. Patient should be encouraged to participate in physiotherapy to strengthen muscles, improve coordination and correct posture and gait.
- Patient's partner's blood should be tested to know if they have contacted syphilis.
- Every effort should be taken to maintain the patient nutrition and general health.

NEUROCYSTICERCOSIS

Definition

Cysticercosis is the condition which results from encystment of the larvae of *Taenia solium*, the pork tapeworm, in the tissues of the brain.

Epidemiology

Neurocysticercosis is the most common parasitic disease of the CNS and one of the most frequent neurological disorder in several countries of Latin America, Africa and Asia.

- Its relavance is related to socioeconomic factors and feeding habits.
- It is almost unnoticed in Muslims as the *Quran* prohibits the consumption of pork.
- It is endemic in areas where pork is massively consumed.
- In Asia this condition is a common disease, but it's prevalence is still underestimated.
- Because of lack of diagnostic facilities in rural areas, where the reported cases only represent the tip of the ice-berg.
- CNS involvement occurs in 50 to 70 percent of all cases.

Pathogenesis

Life cycle of *T. solium* (pork tapeworm) (Fig. 9.1)

T. solium is one of the 30 different types of cestodes that infect man. All have complex life cycles that require at least two hosts. In the case of *T. solium* humans are the only definite host. Whereas both humans and pigs may act as intermediate hosts.

The tapeworm vesicular stage is found in drinking water, unwashed vegetables, contaminated food, undercooked meat, etc. Human who consumes raw or undercooked meat from infected

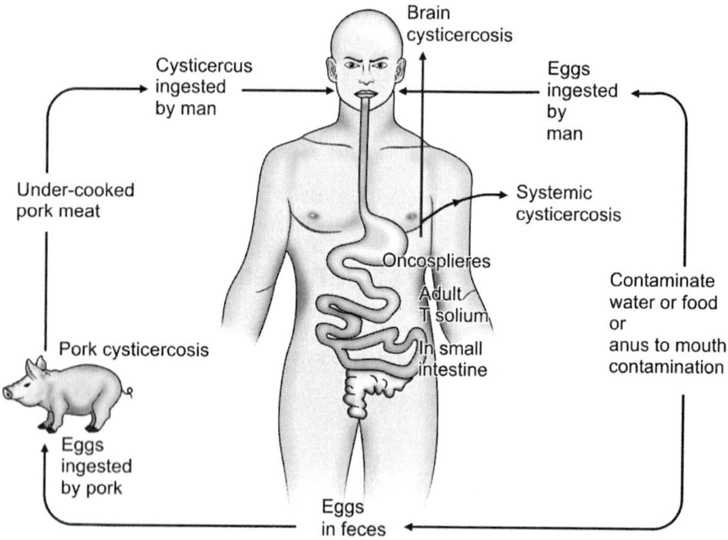

Fig. 9.1: Life cycle of *Taenia solium*

animals can become contaminated and the adult tapeworm develops in the human intestine as the man is definite host. It remains attached to the bowel wall with the aid of its suckers and hooks. Everyday four to five gravid proglottides are detached from the distal end of the body of the worm and are excreted in feces. Each proglottide contain thousands of eggs which can remain viable for long time in water, soil and vegetation.

When pig nourishes the food contaminated with feces containing *T. solium* eggs, the eggs lose their coat liberating oncospheres (embryos) that in turn cross the bowel wall enter the bloodstream and are carried to the muscles and other tissues of the host where larvae (cysticerci) develop. When this meat is ingested by human the larvae evaginate in the small intestine and attach to the bowel wall. It is unusual for a man to be infested with more than one *T. solium* at a time. Man can also act as an intermediate host for *T. solium*. After ingesting its egg the embryos liberated and cysticercosis develop (as described in pig).

The two main sources from which human acquire cysticercosis are:

1. Ingestion of food contaminated with *T. solium* eggs.
2. Anus to mouth contamination in individuals harboring the adult parasite in the intestine. First one is the most common one.

Pathology

Cysticerci may be found in cerebral cortex, basal ganglia, subarachnoid space or ventricular space or spinal cord. Apart from the diversity in the number, location, size and shape of parasite, the inflammatory reaction around cysticerci usually induces multiple changes. Composed of lymphocytes plasma cells and eosinophils, it is usally associated with edema and reactive gliosis. It's intensity varies with stage of the cysticercus. The stages of development are, vesicular stage, colloidal stage, granular stage and calcified stage.

Signs and Symptoms

Most common clinical manifestations are:

1. Seizures: 50 to 80 percent patient with parenchymal brain cyst or calcification will have seizures, less common in the other forms of disease.

2. Focal neurological signs:
   - Pyramidal tract signs
   - Sensory deficits
   - Cerebellar ataxia
   - Signs of brainstem dysfunction
   - Involuntary movement
3. Increased intracranial pressure
4. Hydrocephalus
5. Encephalitis
   - Clouding of consciousness
   - Diminition of visual activity
   - Headache
   - Vomiting
   - Papilledema
6. Psychotic reactions
7. Diffuse muscle involvement may result in psuedohypertrophic myopathy. Swelling and hypertrophy of muscle.

Diagnosis

- CT scan
- MRI
- Immunological tests for anticysticercus antibodies in serum saliva and CSF.
- Stool for ova, cyst, fragments of parasite.

Therapy

Before the treatment the viability of cyst and location of parasite is to be confirmed. Treatment consists of:
1. Symptomatic
2. Specific anticysticercus agents
3. Surgical treatment.

Drugs

1. Praziquantel 25 mg/kg every 2 hours per day
   or
2. Albendazole 15 mg/kg per month

The above drugs (1) and (2) are given under the cover of decadron (corticosteroids) IV (4-8 mg q 8 hourly) to prevent reaction and untoward effects of cysticerci on brain.

Surgical Treatment

1. For patients with hydrocephalus secondary to cysticercosis ventricular shunt is done.
2. Freely mobile ventricular cysts may be removed by surgical excision or endoscopic aspiration.

Nursing Care

- Observe patient's condition, vital signs, and symptoms of increased intracranial pressure.
- Provide seizures precautions.
- Anticipate behavioral change and observe for it.
- Give health education about the disease condition, cause, treatment and prevention.

Prevention of Cysticercosis

It can be done by:
1. Sanitary implementation
2. Treatment of waste water before irrigation of vegetables
3. Hygienic breeding of pigs
4. Compulsory search and treatment of *Taenia solium* carriers
5. Intensive educational programs in populations at risk
6. Following good hygienic habits
7. Pig to be examined and certified before slaughtering
8. Thorough cooking of beef and pork.

NEUROLOGICAL MANIFESTATION DUE TO HIV INFECTION

AIDS is a acronym for the acquired immunodeficiency syndrome. The virus which causes AIDS is known as human immunodeficiency virus (HIV). It belongs to a unique family of viruses known Retroviruses and is endowed with two important properties viz., mutability and latency. At present two types of serotypes of HIV are recognised as HIV-1 and HIV-2.

Sources of Infection

HIV can be transmitted by contact to infected blood or other body fluids. Body fluids which can transmit HIV include the following:
- blood
- vaginal and cervical secretion
- semen

- cerebrospinal fluid
- synovial—pleural fluids, peritoneal, pericardial, secreted from wounds.

Other fluids listed below which unless containing visible blood have not been associated with the transmission of HIV. They are feces, urine, saliva, tears, nasal secretions, sweat, breast milk, and vomitus. So the blood is the single most important route of potential transmission of HIV infection.

Transmission can take place by

1. Sexual intercourse
2. Perinatal transmission
3. Contact with blood and blood products
4. Unscreened blood transfusion
5. Infected needles and syringes while receiving injections or donating blood.

HIV is not transmitted through mere touch, kissing, or even through insects.

Pathophysiology of HIV (Fig. 9.2)

This virus suppresses the immune system of the body. The immune system of human body has many factors which work together to

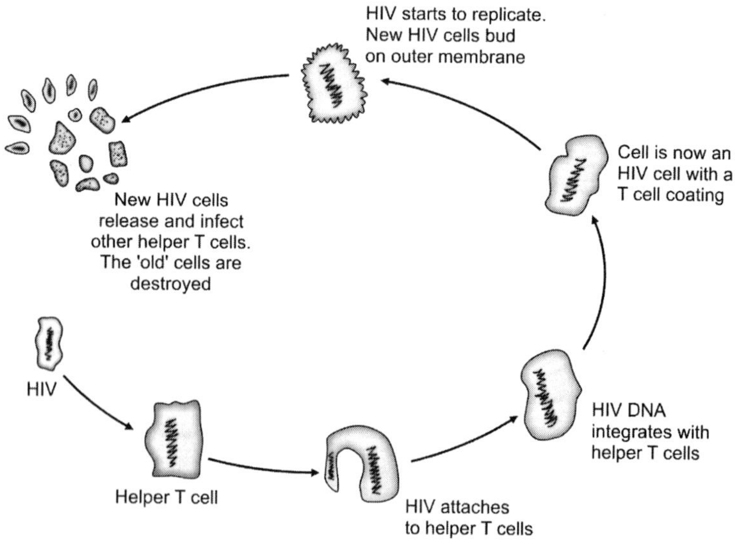

Fig. 9.2: HIV acting on the T_4 cells in human body

produce immunity against the infections, the body feces. White blood cells in blood is one group of cells work to produce immunity. WBCs also have different types of cells and the 'T' lymphocytes are the mediator cells of the body. They are involved in the cell mediated immune system. They protect the body against viral infections and, also against cancer cells. These 'T' cells contain, surface markers or receptors referred to as clusters of differentiation (CE). All mature 'T' cells contain CD2, CD3, CD5 and CD7. Helper 'T' cells contain CD4. So they are called T_4 cells. When a person get infected with the HIV, the HIV attach to T_4 cells. The DNA of HIV integrates with the T_4 cells. Later the HIV becomes the cell itself with T_4 cell covering.

In the later stage HIV starts to replicate new HIV cell buds on the outer membrane (i.e. of T_4 cell membrane). The cell membrane breaks and the multiplied HIV cells (virus) come out to attack other T_4 cells. This process continues to destroy the T_4 cells, to cause the immune deficiency in human body.

Normal count of T_4 cells in human body ranges from 600 to 1200 mm^3. But in persons infected with HIV the count is decreased even up to 50 mm^3 when it becomes less than 200 mm^3 the active symptoms of infection starts.

Clinical Manifestation

The clinical spectrum of infection related to HIV, AIDS range from an asymptomatic state to the severe immunosuppression and related opportunistic diseases associated with the infection. Most individuals are asymptomatic following infection. Approximately 20 percent of them develop fever, myalgia, lethargy, rash, enlarged lymph nodes, sorethroat, nausea after 2 to 4 weeks of infection. These symptoms may last for 1 week though the lethargy can present longer.

During asymptomatic period transmission of virus can occur. The average time before symptoms appear is 10 to 12 years. However, this time is also extremely variable. Some individuals become symptomatic within 5 years of infection and others may not become ill for as long as 12 years.

As the disease progress, some infected individuals develop persistent generalized lymphadenopathy. This also can prolong for years.

Next is the last stage when constitutional symptoms are in the absence of any known underlying cause. This stage can be manifested by:

- cyclical fever,
- night sweats,
- diarrhea, fatigue,
- anorexia, weight loss,
- oral hairy leukoplakia, and
- AIDS dementia complex,
  Candidiasis is also an important predictor of disease progression.

Neurological Manifestation

HIV infection of central nervous system produces dementia, myelopathy and peripheral neuropathy. As many as 80 percent individuals infected with HIV develop neurological manifestations, out of which 10 percent may develop the symptoms in the first stage of the disease itself. The neurological manifestation can be under the headings of

1. Cryptococcal meningitis
2. Cerebral toxoplasmosis
3. CNS tuberculosis
4. Neurosyphilis
5. Pyogenic meningitis
6. Herpes zoster.

Signs and Symptoms

Signs and symptoms can be according to the stages and the opportunistic organism and area of body affected. But common symptoms are:

- Fever
- Lethargy
- Diarrhea
- Weight loss
- Vomiting
- Which do not respond to the usual drugs.

Opportunistic Diseases Due to HIV-AIDS

As HIV infection progresses, the immune system becomes increasingly more compromised and less functional. Numerous infections, a variety of cancers and wasting, result from this impairment. Some of the conditions are—pneumocystis carinii pneumonia. Kaposi's sarcoma (skin cancer).

Diagnostic Studies

- Antibody ELISA—(enzyme linked immunosorbent assay)
- Western blot
- Antigen
- Cell-culture
- Lymphocyte number
- T_4-T_8 lymphocyte counts.

Management

Asymptomatic HIV positive individuals need close medical supervision. The T_4 cells are usually monitored every 3 to 4 months. Although there is no cure for HIV infection, drugs like

1. Zidovudine
2. Didanosine
3. Dideoxycytidine
4. Deoxythymidine
5. Acyclovir, can be used to decrease the speed of infections and decrease the manifestations also. These drugs can also help the person to increase the lifespan.

Nursing Management

1. Symptomatic
2. Prevention of transmission to others
3. Holistic approach as the patient and family face many social, psychological and financial problems associated with stigma attached to the disease.

Symptomatic management can be under the headings of

- Control of fever/treat fever
- Control or treat the nausea vomiting
- Control or treat diarrhea
- Control or treat rashes
- Control or treat respiratory tract infection
- Control or treat the neuroinfection
- Control or treat the neurosymptoms
- Control or treat herpes zoster
- Control and treat the nosocomial infection.

Prevention of Transmission to Other Individuals

Prevention of infection is achieved by

- Barrier nursing.
- Disposal of waste material in an appropriate method with use of 1 percent sodium hypochloride solution for disinfection of any body fluid.
- Solid waste like sanitary pad, dressing materials to be burnt.
- Use only disposable syringes and needles while nursing these patients.
- Used linen to be soaked in sodium hypochloride solution for a minimum duration of 30 minutes.
- Prevent the infected individual from sexual intercourse to the spouse if the spouse is not infected.

Holistic Approach

This holistic approach can be achieved in different strategies.

a. For the patient
    - Help the patient to come out of fear.
    - Develop self-confidence in patient so that the will overcomes the feeling of loss.
    - Crises intervention can be used to help the patient to overcome the grief.
    - Help the patient to ventilate the past events which can overcome the feeling of guilt and depression.
    - Anxiety to be managed by antidepressant drugs.
    - Patient can be referred to guidance clinic if needed.
    - The guidance clinic can assist the patient to get place for rest of his life.
    - This clinic can give him financial help/security.
    - This placement can give him social security but the stigma attached to the institution can cause all psychological problems get triggered.
    - This can be managed only with continuous holistic approach of the managing team.

b. For the family members
    Give them the knowledge about the disease, progress, mode of transmission, course of illness.

Postexposure Prophylaxis

If any individual gets a needle prick while nursing a patient in confirmed HIV infection, a course of prophylaxis can be given to prevent the infection to the individual. The drugs given as prophylaxis are:

1.	Tab Azidothymidine (AZT) Tab Lanuvudinine	200 mg tds with 150 mg BD	4 weeks
2.	Azodothymidine with Lanuvudinine		4 weeks
3.	Tab Duovir	1 tab BD	4 weeks

Blood should be investigated regularly. Follow-up should be at 6 weeks, 12 weeks, and every 6 months later. All these produce side-effects like severe nausea, vomiting and diarrhea.

Some questions which can arise from the patient and family members:

1. **Is HIV transferable?**

Ans. Yes it is.

2. **What are modes of transmission?**

Ans. Sexual intercourse, direct contact with the body fluids of infected person to interrupted skin.

3. **Can mere touch or kiss transmit the disease?**

Ans. No, it is not transmitted through mere handshake, kiss or touch.

4. **Can any one share the toilet used by the individual who is infected with HIV?**

Ans. Yes, it can be used, but only after properly cleaning and disinfecting the toilet.

5. **Can the individual infected with HIV marry?**

Ans. Yes, but only after explaining to the spouse and pregnancy should be avoided as the child will be infected.

6. **Is there any definite treatment for HIV?**

Ans. No, only symptomatic treatment is available. But some drugs can slow down the speed of disease progress.

7. **How long the patient can live after getting infected?**

Ans. He can live up to 12 to 13 years after infection. But few months after the clinical symptoms manifested, life can be prolonged these days as drugs are available to slow down the progression of illness.

8. **Do the individuals show the symptoms soon after they are infected?**

Ans. Surely not—may be asymptomatic even upto 10 to 12 years. They may show the symptoms after 5 years also.

9. **Can the individual infect others when he/she is asymptomatic?**

Ans. Yes he/she can transmit disease while he/she is asymptomatic also.

10. **Is there any vaccination available to prevent HIV/AIDS?**

Ans. So far it is not available. Many works are being carriedout to find a suitable medicine.

11. **How soon after exposure to HIV should get the treatment?**

Ans. Preferably with one to two hours, but other studies suggest it can be started within 24 to 36 hours after the exposure. Early treatment will definitely lessen the severeity of the symptoms and delay the onset of illness.

12. **How long the treatment to be continued?**

Ans. If the patient can tolerate usual course is for 4 weeks.

13. **Is there any side-effect for these drugs?**

Ans. It can cause nausea, vomiting, tiredness, jaundice, kidney stones, etc.

14. **After the treatment how often these individuals should go for follow-up and blood investigations ?**

Ans. Present day advice is to go for follow-up every six months.

Here the discussion of nursing management stops, for time being as it is a burning issue of the healthcare settings, and the researches are on going, there may be changes in the above mentioned discussion frequently so the nurses are to update their knowledge every now and then.

UNIVERSAL PRECAUTIONS TO PREVENT HIV TRANSMISSION IN HEALTHCARE SETTINGS (Published by WHO)

INFECTION CONTROL PRECAUTIONS

- TO PREVENT INJURIES FROM NEEDLES AND OTHER SHARP INSTRUMENTS
  i. Never bend, break or recap disposable needles, but dispose of them immediately with the attached syringe in a thick

cardboard, glass, heavy plastic or metal container. These should be located as close as is practical to the area in which the needles are used.

ii. Place disposable sharp instruments in a thick cardboard, glass, heavy plastic or metal container immediately after use. When full, seal the container carefully and burn or burry in a hygienically controlled sanitary landfill.

iii. Place reusable sharp instruments (e.g. needles, scalpels, etc.) in a glass, heavy plastic or metal container immediately after use. Wear thick gloves to carefully clean needles and all other sharp instruments (and syringes) before disinfection or sterilization.

iv. Avoid unnecessary handling of contaminated sharp instruments, including needles.

- TO PREVENT EXPOSURE OF OPEN WOUNDS AND MUCOUS MEMBRANES

i. Cover broken skin or open wounds with watertight dressings.

ii. Wash hands with water and soap immediately after any contact with blood or other body fluids.

iii. Specimens of blood and other body fluids should be placed in containers with secure lids to prevent leakage during transportation. Avoid contamination of the outer surface of the container.

iv. Wear suitable gloves when expecting exposure to blood or body fluids and when handling blood specimens.

v. Linen soiled with blood and other body fluids should be transported in leak-proof bags, or folded with the soiled part inside. It should be washed in hot water with detergent.

vi. During assistance at childbirth, the nurse may be exposed to extensive amounts of blood. Planning for childbirth in the hospital or in the home should include obtaining gloves, aprons, soap and water.

vii. Wear protective glasses when blood splashes are expected, such as during major surgery, childbirth or dental procedures.

viii. Mouth-to-mouth suction of newborns should be replaced with mechanical or electric suction devices.

ix. Mouth pipetting should be replaced by mechanical pipetting in all laboratories handling blood and other body fluids.

x. Resuscitation bags should be made available in health care settings in which resuscitation is likely to be needed.

- PREVENTING HIV TRANSMISSION VIA CONTAMINATED INSTRUMENTS
  i. All reusable instruments must be cleaned and disinfected or sterilized between use.
  ii. Disposable equipment must be used only once and then appropriately discarded, i.e. burnt or buried.
  iii. Promote oral medication rather than medication by injection when possible; if clients prefer injections, explain why oral medication is preferable.
  iv. Teach patients to avoid injections and skin-piercing carried out by practitioners who do not sterilize their equipment.
- PREVENTING HIV TRANSMISSION VIA TRANSFUSION OF HIV-CONTAMINATED BLOOD OR BLOOD PRODUCTS
  i. All blood for transfusion should be tested for markers of HIV infection. In areas where testing is not feasible, blood transfusions should only be given when absolutely necessary, to treat a life-threatening condition.
  ii. Where possible, replace blood transfusions by other suitable intravenous fluids, e.g. dextrose and/or dextran 70 or Ringer's solutions.
  iii. For patients who are anemic, the cause of anemia should be sought and treated. It is better to prevent the cause of anemia (hookworm, malaria or malnutrition) than to give transfusions.
- PREVENTING HIV TRANSMISSION FROM HIV-CONTAMINATED ORGAN OR TISSUE TRANSPLANT OR SEMEN DONATION
  i. Test all donors for HIV antibody prior to any donation.
- SPILLS OF BLOOD OR OTHER BODY FLUIDS ON SURFACES (e.g. TABLE, FLOOR)
  i. Remove blood or other body fluids with paper towels or old newspapers. Take care not to get blood on the hands, i.e. wear gloves where possible. Cloth towels may be used, but will then be contaminated and must be handled as soiled linen.
  ii. Wash surface with hot water and soap.
  iii. Decontaminate with intermediate or low-level disinfectant, e.g. sodium hypochloride.

- DISPOSAL OF WASTE
  i. Liquids, such as blood, can be flushed into a sanitary sewer or pit latrine.
  ii. Solid waste, for example, blood-soaked dressings, sanitary pads and napkins, placentas or tissue biopsy specimens should be burnt or carefully buried.

Caution: Avoid placing these materials in open dumps to which animals and children have access, and avoid burying materials where there is a possibility of their being dug up or where they might contaminate water sources.

UNIVERSAL PRECAUTIONS TO PREVENT HIV TRANSMISSION

OTHER SELECTED NERVOUS SYSTEM INFECTIONS

1. *Disease*: Creutzfeldt Jakob disease
   Organism: Caused by a prion
   Description /Course:
   - Spongiform encephalopathy characterized by progressive dementia, dysarthria, spastic weakness of limbs, myoclonic jerks and seizures
   - 10 to 30 years is the incubation period
   - Usually occurs in fifth or sixth decade
   - Vascular or spongy like appearance of brain tissue
   - Death is the final outcome.

   Diagnosis: Confirmed by brain biopsy.
   Treatment: Supportive.
2. *Disease*: Herpes zoster
   Organism: Herpes virus varicella zoster

   Description/Course:
   - Latent virus from an attack of chickenpox that remains latent in the sensory ganglia.
   - When the host defenses fail, the virus multiplies within the sensory ganglia and is then transported down the sensory nerve and released to the vesicles at the nerve endings.
   - It involves the dorsal root ganglia and follows the sensory distribution of dermatome.
   - Illness starts with severe pain in the distribution of the nerve roots, often around the trunk or above the eyes in the case of ophthalmic herpes.

- First red patches appear on the skin. It changes to papules → vesicles → pustules → scabs.
- It may attack the ophthalmic branch of the trigeminal nerve and cause scarring of the eyes.
- In geniculate herpes the vesicles develop in the ear and there is often facial paralysis and deafness.

Diagnosis
- Based on clinical findings and vesicles occurring 2 to 5 days after pain.
- Pain along the peripheral nerve.

Treatment: A cyclovir 800 mg, 5 times a day for 7 to 10 days, isolation not required.

3. *Disease:* Poliomyelitis

   Organism: Caused by one or three polio viruses, Type 1, 2 or 3

   Description/course:
   - Attacks the motor cells of the anterior horn cells of the spinal cord.
   - Severity varies from mild limb paralysis to death from paralysis of respiratory muscles.
   - Virus enters by way of the gastrointestinal tract.
   - Spread through contact with feces and pharyngeal secretions from infected persons.

   Diagnosis: Based on clinical findings and isolation of the viruses.
   Treatment: Supportive care may need ventilatory support. They require extensive rehabilitation. Modern vaccination has made the disease a clinical rarity.

4. *Disease*: Tetanus

   Organism: Caused by *Clostridium tetani*

   Description/Course:
   - Spreads through horse and cattle feces that contaminates soil.
   - Enters human body from penetrating and crush wounds.
   - Produces three exotoxins that attack the spinal cord and cranial nerves.
   - Causes severe muscle spasms, extreme sensitivity to stimuli and convulsions.
   - Death may occur from asphyxia.

   Diagnosis: Based on the history and clinical findings.
   Treatment: Administration of antitoxin and supportive care.

Immunoglobin 250 units IM single dose is given usually.

5. *Disease:* Herpes simplex encephalitis

   Organism: Caused by herpes simplex virus type I

   Description/Course:

   - Virus type I is responsible for the common herpatic lesions on oral mucosa is sometime produces acute encephalitis in adult. The reason is not known.
   - This is severe life-threatening illness. Death occurs in 70 to 80 percent cases if treatment is not given before the patient becomes comatosed.
   - Symptoms include fever, nausea, vomiting, headache, confusion, stupor, focal deficits. Some patient also have symptoms of temporal lobe, limbic system, deficits such as olfactory and gustatory, hallucination, anosmia, TLE, etc.
   - Cerebral edema and hemorrhage causes abrupt increase in ICP and cause temporal and brainstem herniation.

   Diagnosis: Virus difficult to isolate early, CSF analysis MRI, CT are carried out and detection of viral DNA is important step in early diagnosis.

   Treatment: Acyclovir (zoviax) and supportive treatment.

10

Cerebrovascular Accidents

STROKE

When the blood supply to the brain is seriously disturbed spontaneously (i.e. not due to trauma or to surgical ligation of cerebral vessels), we speak of a cerebrovascular accident or stroke.

Neurons depend upon constant supply of O_2 which is carried in bloodstream. If the blood supply to brain is interrupted even for a few seconds, damage to neurons occur.

Definition

A definition of stroke by WHO 1971 is 'A focal neurological deficit due to a local disturbance in blood supply to the brain. Its onset is usually abrupt but may extend over a few hours or longer.'

Incidence

1. Stroke is a frequent cause of death.
2. The incidence increases with age. Mainly people between 40 to 60 years are affected more.
3. Brain infarct or stroke occurs 30 percent more frequently in men than in women.

Types of Strokes

Stroke can be divided into two major types

1. *Ischemic stroke:* Where the supply of blood to a part of the brain suddenly becomes inadequate for the brain to function. It accounts for 85 percent.
2. *The hemorrhagic stroke:* Where a blood vessel ruptures and blood rushes either through the brain tissue destroying it (cerebral hemorrhage) or outside the brain itself into the subarachnoid

space (subarachnoid hemorrhage) sometimes both these occurs at the same time. It accounts for 15 percent of all strokes.

Causes of Ischemic Strokes (Fig. 10.1)

The term ischemic mean a shortage of blood supply. It occurs due to:

a. *Cerebral thrombosis:* A blood vessel in the brain may be diseased, the usual disease being atheroma where a plaque of hard fatty degenerative nature forms on the inner wall of the artery. This impedes blood flow and as a result a clot forms, which increases in size, finally blocking the vessels completely. This is called cerebral thrombosis.
b. *Cerebral embolism:* A clot may have formed in a vessel outside the brain, such as one of the big vessels in the neck or thorax, of course in the heart itself. Pieces of this clot may break off and are moved by the bloodstream until they lodge in a vessel too small to allow them to pass further. When they block the vessel, the result is the same as a cerebral thrombosis. But this process is called cerebral embolism. The clot responsible is called embolus.
c. *Cerebral ischemia:* One of the important blood vessels supplying brain may (carotid or vertebral) be so diseased that it is markedly narrowed. Under normal circumstances enough blood may pass through to nourish the brain. But if something unusual happens like thromboembolism thrombose in the artery or emboli from elsewhere may reduce blood flow transiently till it recovers spontaneously. If it resolves within 24 hours, it is called TIA (transient ischemic attack). It is very transient and the disability rapidly clears up. Patient experiences a mild transient interruption of neurological function such as tingling, weakness

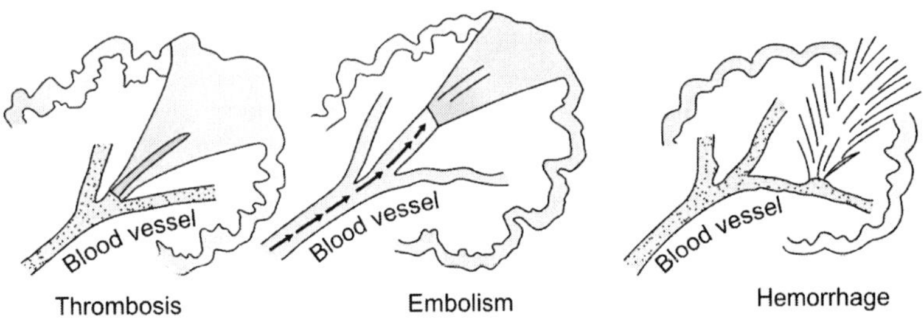

Fig. 10.1: Types of stroke

in one extremity, muddle speech which disappear as quickly as symptoms appear. Thus there is a spectrum of cerebral ischemia from TIA, to complete infarct.

Effect of Cerebral Ischemia

In complete thrombosis a cone-shaped area of the brain rendered short of blood and some of the cells die and never recover. Others are temporarily knocked out of action but recover as other vessels take over the task of the one that is blocked. This area is known as a cerebral infarct and the process as cerebral infarction.

In transient ischemic attack the cells are not deprived of blood and O_2 for long enough for them to die. So they are only temporarily knocked out of action and blood flow is restored and infarct does not occur.

Causes of Hemorrhagic Stroke

Cerebral hemorrhage: Here the wall of the cerebral vessel ruptures and the blood rushes into and through the brain destroying the brain tissues by its sheer force. This is called cerebral hemorrhage. It usually results due to:

- weakness in the vessel wall (athiromas),
- high BP,
- age of 55 or more,
- cerebral aneurysms and
- arteriovenus malformations.

Due to cerebral hemorrhage intracerebral hematomas may form which acts like space occupying lesions and needs surgical intervention.

Risk Factors for Stroke

There are many factors predisposed for stroke, which include:

1. Hypertension,
2. Diabetes mellitus
3. High serum cholesterol level
4. Cigaret smoking
5. Obesity
6. Cardiac disease
7. Use of oral contraceptives
8. Hereditary predisposition.

In younger victims various factors include

- Congenital abnormalities such as cerebral aneurysm
- Arteriovenus malformations (angiomas)
- Premature atherosclerosis
- Embolus/discection of arteries.

Pathophysiology

Stroke can be a quick devastating event because of brain's circulatory and metabolic needs for survival. The brain uses 15 percent of the cardiac output and consumes 20 percent of O_2 supply available for entire body.

Brain does not have any reserves. Hence when blood vessel is occluded over 6 mts the area involved undergoes necrosis which is surrounded by area which is still viable but nonfunctional. This is called ischemic penumbra. With the cerebral infarction, there is edema which results in increased ICP and herniation.

In hemorrhagic stroke the blood is freed into the surrounding cerebral parenchyma creating a hematoma. The hematoma displaces and compresses the adjacent cerebral tissue and ischemic cellular response and cerebral edema occurs resulting in increased ICP. A major ICH can cause midline displacement and herniation syndromes and has a high mortality rate of about 50 percent.

Clinical Manifestation

The result of interruption of blood to the brain may cause temporary or permanent loss of movement, thought, memory, speech, sensation etc. There will be:

- Sudden severe headache
- Numbness, weakness
- Hemiplegia
- Difficulty in speaking or swallowing
- Visual field deficits (homonymous hemianopia—loss of half of the visual field)
- Incoordination of limb or gait
- Impairment of sensation
- Impairment of mental activity
- Impairment of memory and behavior
- Depression.

Symptoms According to the Artery Occluded

Internal Carotid Artery

TIA as warning sign,
After complete occlusion patient becomes:

- unconscious,
- confused,
- hemiplegia and
- hemianesthesia and hemianopia (loss of vision).

If dominent cerebral hemisphere affected expressive and receptive dysphasia will occur.

Anterior Cerebral Artery

- Lower limbs are affected severely
- Dysphasia and apraxia (forgetting simple learned activities)
- Urinary incontinence.

Middle Cerebral Artery

- Hemiplegia
- Dysphasia is common.

Posterior Cerebral Artery

- Hemiplegia
- Blindness
- Visual agnosia (inability to recognize)
- Spontaneous pain and confusion
- Recovery is usually poor and mortality rate is high.

Basilar Artery

Varieties of symptoms occur such as:

- Disturbance of balance and hearing
- Motor and sensory loss
- Loss of consciousness
- Cheyne-Stokes respiration
- Small and fixed pupils
- Tremors and dysphagia.

Manifestation of Hemisphere Involvement

When nondominant hemisphere is involved hemiplegia and hemianopia occurs on opposite side, so patient may develop anosognosia—(a failure to recognize the affected side).

In right-handed people, the left hemisphere is dominant. So when left hemisphere is damaged, the speech is affected. The usual difficulty is in understanding verbal or written instructions but demonstration is effective. And in left hemisphere damage, logic and ideas are also disturbed. Damage to the right perietal lobe may result in difficulties with perception, orientation and also to recognize the familiar faces and objects.

Diagnosis

Some important investigations performed in relation to stroke patient are:
- History and examination, CT head plain, rarely MRI
- Cerebral angiography (optional)
- Lumbal puncture (optional, during recovery phase to look for chronic meningitis
- Other routine investigation, i.e. urine, cholesterol, and triglyceride levels in blood.

Treatment of Stroke

Treatment is done under two headings:

Medical Management

It depends upon patient's age and condition of patient and neurologist preference it includes
a. Close observation and monitoring of hemodynamic parameters.
b. Management of increased ICP control due to cerebral edema mannitol 100 mg IV 6-hourly given.
c. Anticoagulation therapy (except for hemorrhage stroke) heparin 5000 units S/C 8 or 6-hourly for cerebrovenous thrombosis and for cardioembolic stroke.
d. For patients with ischemic stroke and DVT prophylaxis injection heparin 5000 units twice a day to be given.

In Ischemic Stroke

1. Aspirin 325 mg/od given orally.
2. Trental 300 mg IV 12-hourly in the acute phase for initial 3 to 5 days, later trental tablets 400 mg tds may be given for a month.
3. Some people believe in giving low molecular heparin in ischemic stroke.
4. In cerebral venus thrombosis low dose heparin as 5000 IV subcutaneous 8-hourly given in most of the centers for 7 days. Later converted to oral anticoagulant (warfarin).

Surgical Treatment

Carotid endarterectomy or extracranial graft may be done for the patients with narrowing of the extracranial artery. A bypass grafting may be of value for the patient with the intracranial occlusion, such as of the internal carotid or middle cerebral artery. For patients who have an identified thrombus, a thrombectomy may be done to restore circulation.

Complications of Stroke

- Deep vein thrombosis
- Pulmonary embolism
- Aspiration pneumonia
- Spasticity
- Joint contractures with associated pain
- Poststroke depression
- Recurrent stroke
- Bedsore
- Hospital acquired sepsis
- UTI.

NURSING MANAGEMENT

Nursing management of patient with stroke varies according to specific stroke syndrome and neurological and functional deficits. The areas to be considered are:

1. Care during acute phase
2. Maintenance of body functions and prevention of complication
3. Psychological needs

4. Rehabilitation
5. Discharge planning and continuity of care.

Nursing Care during Acute Phase (First 24–48 hours)

Early treatment and nursing care is recognized as a key factor in optimizing outcomes. Patient may be cared in ICU or special acute care unit. During acute stage patient may be unconscious/ altered sensorium. Patient may be unable to maintain his/her own airway due to loss of consciousness, damage to brain tissue and raised ICP inhibits the respiratory center resulting in inadequate ventilation. So—

1. Maintain clear airway for adequate ventilation and to prevent hypoxia
   - Oxygen therapy to be started soon after receiving the patient be sure that it is adequately humidified.
   - In severe cases artificial ventilators may be used if needed.
   - Position the patient to facilitate drainage of oropharyngeal secretions, turn the patient from side-to-side every 2 hours.
   - Suctioning to be done as and when necessary.
   - Elevate the head end of the bed to 30° angle.
   - Maintain patient head in neutral position.
   - Provide for chest physical therapy every 3-hourly.
   - Monitor vital signs.
2. Observe and record her vital signs and neurological status as frequently as necessary.
   - Observe and record the rate, rhythm and depth of respirations frequently to monitor any changes in patient condition
   - Pulse: a slowing pulse rate indicates rising ICP.
   - Temperature: hyperpyrexia could indicate damage to hypothalamus.
   - Level of consciousness: response to verbal/painful stimuli to detect stability, improvement or deterioration in her condition.
   - Pupil size and reaction to light: unequal pupils, dilatation or sluggish response indicates pressure on the oculomotor nerve.
   - Limb movement: spontaneous response to painful stimuli/ abnormal movements. Note any paralysis and type (spastic or flaccid) or paresis.

   Initial observation will provide a base line for future recordings and any changes should be immediately informed.

3. Draw the blood for necessary investigations like ABG (arterial blood gas) level and sodium and potassium levels, group and cross matching. Keep the IV line patent, wait for the blood investigation report, especially electrolytes and urea and connect to IV fluids accordingly. Patient may also be given I/V mannitol or heparin.
   a. Care of the patient while on mannitol drip:
      - Patient may develop electrolyte imbalance so first 4 days blood to be sent for biochemical investigations every day. Later every 3 to 4 days.
      - Intake and output chart to be maintained.
      - If patient is conscious increase oral fluids.
   b. Care of the patient while on heparin administration:
      - Monitor neurological signs for evidence of deterioration and increased ICP.
      - Monitor coagulation studies and maintain therapeutic range using INR parameters.
      - Monitor for bleeding at catheter site and from urine, stool, GI tract or mouth, note evidence of bruising easily.
4. Provide necessary personal hygiene as per the patient condition.
5. Skin care to be taken to prevent bedsores.
6. Monitor indwelling catheter.
7. Provide passive exercises to all joints 4 times daily.
8. When the patient is in altered sensorium:
   - Maintain nothing by mouth status
   - Swallow studies to be done to evaluate swallowing function before oral intake is tried.
   - Ryles tube feedings to be given to compensate nutritional needs.
9. Assess type of communication deficit present and develop appropriate methods for communication.
10. Use strict aseptic technique while carrying out any procedures for the patient.

Postacute Phase

After return to consciousness, coughing and swallowing reflexes may be impaired for sometime. So—

1. *Maintain clear airway to prevent hypoxia*
   - Continue to provide humidified oxygen.
   - Continue to provide care associated with specific needs, such as tracheostomy or aided ventilation as required.

- Offer explanations and reassurance to alleviate patient's anxieties. Breathing will be easier if she is calm and relaxed.
- Continue to observe and record vital signs.
- Encourage deep breathing exercises.
- Chest physiotherapy to be given if needed.

2. *Maintain safe environment:* There is a risk of injury because of unfamiliar environment, neurological dysfunction and impaired movement. Patient remains at risk for further cerebral damage if hemorrhage recurs.
   - Padded cot–sides may be used to prevent her from falling.
   - Change her position frequently in order to prevent pressure sores. Provide aids if required to assist in the prevention of pressure sores and foot drop.
   - Maintain hygienic and aseptic procedures in order to reduce the risk of infection.
3. *Establish effective communication*
   - Stimulate the patient by verbal communication and by touch.
   - Assess type of communication deficit present.
   - Approach the patient from the unaffected side.
   - Speak clearly and in simple sentence, use gestures as necessary.
   - Observe for any specific difficulties which impair communication. Expressive/receptive dysphasia, impaired vision/ or hearing and find the best methods to overcome these.
   - The patient attempt to communicate should be supported.
4. *Encourage mobilization/prevent contractures*
   - Position the patient in bed correctly to prevent contractures, relieve pressure and maintain good body alignment, use aids such as pillows, foam pads, splints, to prevent contractures, and to keep in functional position.
   - Provide for range of motion exercises four times a day to prevent joint stiffness and muscle wasting and help in circulation.
   - Encourage the patient to use his unaffected side to exercise his affected limb.
5. *Meeting nutritional needs:* Patient may be having dysphasia and impaired swallowing reflex. May experience nausea/vomiting due to cerebral lesion. Nasogastric feed is given.
   - Feeds should be given in small amount at frequent intervals.
   - Charting of amount of feed and fluids should be done to ensure the daily intake is sufficient.

- Observe for the return of coughing and swallowing reflex. Provide adequate nutrition.

6. *Elimination:* Patient may be unable to control bladder and bowel function.
   - Observe for incontinence of urine and feces.
   - Institute bladder and bowel retraining if necessary.
   - Patient may be put on continuous urinary drainage—if so care to be taken to prevent UTI.
7. *Personal hygiene:* Provide assistance to maintain personal hygiene.
8. *Diversion:* Patient is in different environment with changes in normal routine and activities.
   - Encourage contact with other patients and her visitors.
   - Provide suitable diversional therapy in which patient has an interest and is capable of participating.
   - Provide opportunities for the patient to participate in usual religious activities.
   - Provide simple work which she can do at bedside and appreciate her performance.

Psychological Needs

Stroke patients may have emotional lability (exhibits reactions easily or inappropriately, loss of self-control, reduced tolerance to stress, fear, hostility, frustration, withdrawal, isolation and depression).

- Reassure the patient and family.
- Neglect bursts of emotions: Explain to the patient that emotional lability is part of the illness.
- Control the environment and maintain routines as much as possible, remove stimuli that are upsetting.
- Anticipate his need and meet them in time.
- Clarify any misconceptions: Allow the patient to verbalize his feelings.
- Give positive feedback.

Rehabilitation

Rehabilitation begins as soon as the patient is stabilized.

- Encourage the patient to do as much of his or her own personal hygiene as possible which increases independence.

- Teach activities of daily living (ADLS) with respect to ways to compensate for the patient disability. ADLS include dressing, toileting, bathing, eating, gait training, so forth.
- Teach the patient transfer techniques (e.g. bed to chair, chair to bed).
- Encourage family participation.

Discharge Planning and Continuity of Care

1. Stress the importance of follow-up care.
2. Make the patient and family aware of community resources which he/she can utilize for her/his rehabilitation.
3. Depression is common after stroke (been in 40-50% of patients) patient and family need to be prepared for this possibility.
4. Instruct the family as follows:
   - Expect some emotional lability and some degree of brain damage if the patient had a more severe stroke. The patient may have episodes of inappropriate behavior crying/ laughing, temper outbursts, etc. They may be easily confused, forgetful, hostile, uncooperative. Support the patient psychologically.
   - Avoid doing those things for the patient that he can do for himself.
   - Be supportive, optimistic but firm and direct.
   - Install handrails by the toilet and shower and put safety rails on the bed.
   - Encourage the patient to keep active and adhere to exercise program and to remain as self-sufficient as possible.
   - Explain that the patient becomes easily fatigued. See that the patient has scheduled rest periods. Promote sense of progress and improvement.
   - To bring the patient for regular follow-up for blood test for coagulation and INR to adjust drug dosages as they will be discharged on medication of antiplatelets and anticoagulants.

Recovery

The extent of the stroke and pre-existing disease influence the degree of recovery. Most of natural recovery in motor function and speech occurs in the first 3 to 6 months.

Nurses' Responsibilities in Prevention of Strokes

One of the most important aspect of nursing care in stroke patient is the prevention—by identifying at risk individual's and dealing with early predisposing factors such as:

1. Transient ischemic attack
2. Hypertension
3. High blood cholesterol
4. Cigaret smoking
5. Overweight
6. Diabetes
7. Use of contraceptive pills.

This identification and treatment can be for affected patients from recurring the stroke and for general population by the way of health teaching to prevent the occurrence.

CEREBRAL VENOUS THROMBOSIS (CVT)

Cerebral venous thrombosis (CVT) is due to occlusion of cerebral veins and/or sinuses. They have a distinct clinical profile, usually affect young persons, more often females and carry a significant mortality.

Epidemiology

Puerperal CVT may account for 15 to 20 percent of stroke in the younger age. It is the most common cause of stroke in young women in India. Fifty percent of strokes in Indian women are related to pregnancy and the puerperium and 95.5 percent of these are due to CVT (Srinivasan K). In western countries the incidence of CVT related to pregnancy and puerperium varies from 1 in 1666 to 10,000 pregnancies.

Causes of CVT

Recognized causes or predisposing conditions

There are a number of local and regional causes either infective or noninfective. They are:

1. *Infective*
   a. Local causes
      - Direct septic trauma
      - Intracranial infection (abscess, empyema meningitis)

- Regional infections, otitis, tonsillitis, sinusitis, stomatitis, skin infections.

b. General causes
- Bacterial: Septicemia, endocarditis, typhoid, tuberculosis
- Viral: Measles, hepatitis, encephalitis, HIV
- Parasitic: Malaria trichinosis
- Fungal: Aspergillosis.

2. *Noninfective*

a. Local causes
- Head injury
- Neurosurgical operations
- Cerebral infarcts and hemorrhage, tumors
- Infusion into internal jugular vein.

b. General causes
- Gyneco-obstetrics
  i. Pregnancy and puerperium
  ii. Oral contraceptives (estrogen, progestogen)
- Cardiac
  i. Congenital heart diseases
  ii. Cardiac insufficiency
  iii. Pacemaker
- Malignancies
- RBC disorders
  i. Polycythemia
  ii. Thrombocythemia
- Coagulation disorder
  i. Antithrombin III Protein C and Protein S deficiency
  ii. Circulating anticoagulants
  iii. Heparin
- Severe dehydration of any cause
- Digestive cirrhosis
- Others
  i. Androgen therapy
  ii. Parenteral injection, etc.

In puerperium, fibrinogen, platelets and factor VIII increases. Increased plasma viscosity and reduced RBC depermiability favors thrombosis.

Pathology

The lesions follow distinct pattern according to the veins and sinuses involved. Occlusion of the superior sagittal sinus and its tributary veins, is the most common lesion in pregnancy related cases.

Superficial venous system is more frequently affected than deep venous system.

When affected, brain will be swollen, edematous and heavy with a mottled gray cyanotic discoloration of the outer surface. More advanced cases show hemorrhagic infarction. Cerebral infarction results from extension of thrombosis to cerebral veins. Most of the infarcts are hemorrhagic necrotic lesions uneven distribution.

Clinical manifestations depend upon the area affected. As in stroke, patient will have:

- Headache
- Papilledema
- Focal deficits (hemiparesis and hemisensory disturbances are found more frequently than dysphasia or hemianopia)
- Seizures, partial, general, status epilepticus
- Mental changes
- Altered sensorium
- Multiple cranial nerve palsies
- Cerebral incoordination.

Diagnosis

Diagnosis made by

- CT scan
- MRI
- Angiography
- EEG
- CSF examination
- Blood investigations (detail coagulation studies).

Management and nursing care is as written in the case of stroke.

11

Epilepsy

Nerve cells function by discharging small electrical waves. Those discharges arising from the brain can be measured by electro-encephalograph (EEG). If the brain cells suddenly produce a burst of very much larger electrical waves than normal, then an epileptic fit may result. Patients whose brains have a tendency to do it repeatedly are said to suffer from epilepsy.

Definition

Epilepsy is a recurrent/paroxysmal disorder due to abnormal excessive electrical discharge from brain cells resulting in brief, stereotyped episodes with or without loss of consciousness (Dr P Satishchandra).

A single seizure does not constitute epilepsy. The word recurrent is important in the definition. Though the term seizure, convulsions and fits are used synonymously. It is to be noted that not all seizure or convulsions are epileptic, however, *vice versa* is true.

Magnitude of Epilepsy

Recent epidemiological surveys conducted in different parts of India including Bangalore Urban Rural Neuroepidemiological (BURN) study, report a prevalence of 8 per 1000 population of active epilepsy. That means there are approximately 8 million people with epilepsy in India constituting one-fifth of the global epilepsy problem. Prevalence of active epilepsy seems to be 2 to 2.5 times higher in the rural as compared to urban population.

Classification of Epilepsy

The preferred method of classifying seizures is the international classification system was revised in 1981. It is based on the clinical and electroencephalographic (EEG) manifestation. In this system seizures are divided into three major classes:

I. Partial seizures
II. Generalized seizures
III. Unclassified epileptic seizures:
    - Reflex epilepsy
    - Nonepileptic attacks, etc.

I. Partial (Focal, Localized) Seizures

a. Simple partial seizures (no impairment of consciousness)
    - With motor signs
    - With somatosensory or special sensory systems
    - With autonomic symptoms or signs
    - With psychic symptoms.
b. Complex partial seizures (impairment of consciousness)
    - Simple partial onset followed by impairment of consciousness
    - With impairment of consciousness at onset.
c. Partial seizures evolving to secondary generalized seizures
    - Simple partial seizures evolving to generalized seizures
    - Complex partial seizures evolving to generalized seizures
    - Simple partial seizures evolving to complex partial seizures evolving to generalized seizures.

II. Generalized Seizures (Convulsive or Nonconvulsive)

a. Absence seizures
    - Typical absence
    - Atypical absence
b. Myoclonic seizures
c. Clonic seizures
d. Tonic seizures
e. Tonic-clonic seizures
f. Atonic seizures (astatic seizures).

Partial Seizures

The seizures produced as a result of a localized disturbance continued to a small area of the brain. The clinical characteristics depend upon the part of the brain affected. They are divided into three main categories.

1. Simple partial: in which there is no alteration of consciousness.
2. Complex partial: in which consciousness is altered.
3. Partial seizures evolving into secondary generalized seizures.

A. Simple Partial Seizures (SPS)

It occurs due to a focus within a particular part of the brain, usually the motor strip is irritated producing disturbance in function of the affected area of the body. This can occur at any age. Any cortical regions may be affected the most common regions being frontal, and parietal lobes. There will not be loss of consciousness.

Symptoms are:

Motor symptoms

- Clonic movements of limbs or face on one side
- Facial twitching.

Sensory symptoms

- Tingling or numbness or burning or pain
- Electrical shock like sensation
- Simple visual manifestations such as flashes of lights and colors.

This is also called focal seizures. The focal seizures remain isolated but when it spreads to affect the other parts of the body, it is described as Jacksonian fit. Example—the convulsion begin in the fingers of one side, spread to the hand, wrist, forearm, face and finally the lower extremity on the same side of the body and leads to unconsciousness and a generalized seizure.

B. Complex Partial Seizure (CPS)

Most commonly 60 percent originate from temporal lobe where an irritant may produce a characteristic distinctive type of seizures. Thirty percent can also occur from extratemporal regions—frontal cortex.

Clinical features include:

1. Auras, e.g. pins and needles, followed by

2. Altered consciousness
3. Amnesia
4. Automatism: defined as more or less coordinated involuntary motor activity usually followed by amnesia of the event.
   Common examples of automation are lip smacking, chewing, facial grimacing, swallowing movements and patting, picking or rubbing oneself or one's clothing. Patient may appear 'wild eyed' and may speak in jumbled, repetitive phrases if addressed. Temporal lobe seizures generally last from 1 to 4 minutes and are followed by several minutes of postictal confusion.
5. Sudden onset and recovery.

C. Partial Seizures Evolving to Secondarily Generalized Seizures

Both simple partial or complex partial seizures initially start as partial may spread to become generalized. Partial seizure is experienced as aura for few seconds before generalization occurs with complete loss of consciousness.

Primary Generalized Seizures

Primary generalized seizure is defined as an attack in which electrical disturbances involve wide areas of both cerebral hemisphere with no evidence of anatomical or functional focus. Consciousness is impaired from the onset. Motor phenomenon is usually bilateral, more or less symmetrical EEG patterns are bilateral and grossly synchronous.

Absence Seizures

The ILAE (International League Against Epilepsy) divides absence seizure into typical and atypical absence.

a. *Typical absence:* It was previously known as petit mal epilepsy. They occur most often in childhood or adolescence and are almost exclusively idiopathic generalized epilepsy. The attack is characterized by abrupt cessation of activity with a momentary arrest of consciousness lasting about 5 to 10 seconds.
   Due to momentary loss of touch with the surroundings, the child may pauses in conversation, the eyelids may flicker, the head nod, something may be dropped, words or figures may

be repeated and then the child picks up the conversation. Only a close observer realizes that something has been wrong.

The attacks occur very frequently, number of times per hour, or day and are very brief stereotyped without any postictal phenomenon. Eighty percent of absence lasts less than 10 seconds and many hundreds of attacks may occur in a single day. Attack could be easily precipitated by hyperventilation or sometimes by photic stimulation.

b. *Atypical absence* differs from typical absence in clinical manifestations, EEG and etiology. Duration is longer, onset and cessation is not so abrupt. Focal signs are more prominent and include tone changes, clonic jerking automation. It occurs in symptomatic epilepsies and are associated with mental retardation (MR) and other neurological abnormalities.

Absence needs to be differentiated from complex partial seizures since treatment and natural history differs.

Myoclonic Seizures

Myoclonus is defined as sudden brief, jerky contraction of a muscle or group of muscles or organ. It can be single or repetitive varying in severity. Recovery is immediate and patient often says that consciousness is not lost. Sometimes it can preceded a tonic clonic seizures.

Myoclonus can develop at any age, e.g. Wests syndrome, Lennox Gastuat syndrome, Juvenile myoclonic epilepsy, progressive myoclonic epilepsy, etc.

Generalized Tonic Clonic Seizures (GTCS)

Grand mal epilepsy (the seizure that most people associate with epilepsy).

Tonic clonic seizure affects both children and adults and is a common variety of seizure activity. It comprises several distinct stages.

Stage 1. *Aura:* A strange feeling or taste in the mouth.
It is a warning of the impending fit.
Patient places himself in a position of safety.
In many cases warning may not be present.

2. *Sudden loss of consciousness:* If patient is standing, he falls to the ground.

3. *Tonic stage:* It lasts less than a minute.
4. *Clonic stage:* is characterized by rhythmic, muscular contractions of the limbs and stertorous breathing over a period of 30 seconds or longer. After the clonic phase the person is unconscious for about 5 minutes.
5. *Postictal phase:* Confusion and disorientation is common. Patient may complain of headache, generalized muscular aching and fatigue. There is no recollection of the attack.

The seizures may occur at any time of the day or night. Whether the patient is awake or asleep. The attack lasts from 2 to 3 minutes. The frequency of recurrence can vary from hours to weeks, months or years. Sometimes patients may have only tonic seizures or only clonic seizures. At times clonic component could be restricted to only one half of the body. These are known as unilateral seizures.

Atonic Seizures

Atonic seizures may take any form. The classic drop attack (astatic seizures) is clonic seizure in which postural tone is lost resulting in fall to the ground. Sometimes it may be restricted, e.g. nodding of head, bowing movement, sagging at the knee. They are very brief, occur without warning followed by immediate recovery. Usually these are often symptomatic, occur usually with mental retardation.

Unilateral seizure: Nearly one-third of seizures are considered unclassified.

Reflex Epilepsy (Table 11.1)

Reflex epilepsy is unusual form of seizures disorder where the seizures are provoked by a specific external stimulus or event. The stimulus may be television, video games, flickering of light, specific sound, hot water, calculation, reading, exercise, startle, etc.

Nonepileptic Attacks (Table 11.2)

They are also called pseudoseizures or sometimes patients with epilepsy might also has these nonepileptic attacks. Conversion disorder presents either as dissociative symptoms or as a conversion hysteria. Secondary gain is noticed in these patients. It is essential to take an adequate history, both neurological and psychiatric features.

Table 11.1: Triggering factors in reflex epilepsies

1. *Visual stimuli*	2. *Auditory*	3. *Somatosensory*
Patterns Television Video games Eye closure Flickering light	Specific sound Music Specific voice	Tap/touch Hot water epilepsy Tooth brushing
4. *Mental (Thinking)*	5. *Motor*	6. *Other (combination)*
Calculation Problem solving e.g. Chess Arithmetic Card games	Movement (Kinesogenic) Eye movements	Reading Eating Exercise Startle

Table 11.2: Difference between genuine epilepsy and hysterical epilepsy

	Genuine epilepsy	*Hysterical epilepsy*
1. History of fall and injury	Present	Absent
2. Fits when alone/during sleep	Yes	No
3. Movement of the limbs	Regular	Irregular
4. Tongue bite	Yes	No
5. Incontinence of urine and feces	Present	No
6. Inducing an attack by strong suggestion	Not possible	Possible
7. During an attack pupils	Dilated	Normal
8. Automatic arousal	Present	Only after the intervention by others

Status Epilepticus (SE)

Status epilepticus is a fairly common life-threatening emergency in any general hospital. It is defined as a single seizure lasting 30 minutes or longer or as a condition in which seizures recur so frequently that the patient does not completely regain consciousness before having another.

SE occurs at a frequency of about 18 to 24 per 100,000 population per year. The incidence is highest in children and in adults above 60 years of age. Eighty percent SE are of tonic clonic type among patients with long-standing epilepsy. Up to 5 percent of adults and more than 10 percent of children may be expected to have SE over the course of their epilepsy. Anticonvulsant withdrawal in patients with known epilepsy, neuroinfections (including cysticercosis and tuberculosis), trauma are the most common causes for status epilepticus (Dr Arunodaya).

Causes of Epilepsy

Unknown—but suggested causes are:
- Cerebrovascular disorders trauma
- CNS infections
- Systemic diseases, diabetics, high BP, low BP
- Toxic conditions
- Cerebral degenerative diseases
- Tumors of the brain
- Metabolic disorders
- Miscellaneous
  - Drug withdrawal
  - Alcoholism.

In children between 6 months to 5 years the common causes are:
- Febrile convulsions
- Perinatal trauma
- CNS infection, e.g. viral encephalitis
- Systemic disease
  - Cysticercosis
  - TB
- Intracranial lesions
- Miscellaneous
  - Trauma.

Diagnosis

Diagnosis is made from:
1. History
   - Eyewitness account of attack
   - Circumstances
   - Timings
   - Precipitating factors
   - Preictal symptoms
   - Ictal events
   - Postictal symptoms
   - Any injuries associated with seizures
   - Loss of consciousness

2. EEG
3. Laboratory studies
4. X-ray skull
5. CT scan.

Differential diagnosis

- Syncope
- Hysterical seizure
- Others
  - Transient ischemic attacks
  - Confusional state
  - Hypoglycemia
  - Panic attacks.

Medical Management of Epilepsy

- Treatment of the cause factor
- Anticonvulsant drug therapy

If properly prescribed and taken, these drugs will result in control of more than 50 percent of patients with recurring seizures.

For generalized epilepsy—Tab phenobarbitone which is inexpensive and effective is started with a small dose depending upon the age of the patient:

3 years—15 mg single dose bed time

3 to 10 years—30 mg single dose bed time

Above 10 years—60 mg single dose bed time

In adults, it may be given upto 180 mg/day. If attacks are not controlled tab phenytoin is added. Drugs have to be taken for a minimum period of 3 to 5 years after the last fit.

The following are the various antiepileptic drugs that are in use:

Primary drugs are those that are used commonly in various types of epilepsies and are time tested. Various newer drugs (Table 11.3) are used as an add-on therapy. Some of them have been also used as first line drugs. The long-term experience with these drugs are limited.

The following are the first and the second choice of drugs (Table 11.4) in various types of epilepsies and epileptic syndrome. The sequence of choice depends on individual experience, availability of the drug and the cost. There is no significant difference

Table 11.3: Various antiepileptic drugs

Primary drugs	*Newer drugs*
1. Phenobarbitone	1. Lamotrigine
2. Phenytoin	2. Gabapentin
3. Primidone	3. Felbamate
4. Carbamazepine	4. Vigabatrin
5. Ethosuximide	5. Tiagabine
6. Valproate	6. Topiramate
7. Clonazepam	7. Remacemide
8. Clobazam	8. Zonisamide
9. Acetazolamide	9. NMDA receptor antagonist
	10. GABA B receptor antagonist
	11. LO59
	12. Eterobarb

Table 11.4: First and second choice drugs

Seizure types	*First choice*	*Second choice*
Generalized seizure Tonic-clonic, clonic	Valproate Carbamazepine	Phenytoin Lamotrigine Clobazam Vigabatrin Phenobarbitone Acetazolamide Felbamate
Myoclonic epilepsy	Valproate	Clonazepam Piracetam Phenobarbitone Acetazolamide
Absence Lamotrigine	Valproate	Ethosuximide Clonazepam Acetazolamide
Atypical Absences, Atonic, Tonic	Valproate	Lamotrigine Clonazepam Clobazam Phenobarbitone Acetazolamide Felbamate Phenytoin Gabapentine
Partial seizures Simple partial Complex parital Secondarily generalized	Carbamazepine Valproate	Phenytoin Lamotrigine Clobazam Gabapentine Acetazolamide Phenobarbitone Felbamate

in the efficacy of these drugs in various seizure syndromes. The usage is mainly dictated and limited by side effects and the cost.

Surgical Treatment

About 5 percent of patients with epilepsy may be good candidates for surgery. Patients who have not responded to medical management, who have a unilateral focus that will not cause a major neurological deficit if exercised and who had a significant alteration in their quality of life are good candidates.

The purpose of surgery is to locate and exercise as much of the epileptogenic area as possible. Temporal lobectomy is usually done.

Nursing Management of the Patients with Seizures

Nursing management of patients with seizures consists of:

1. Providing accurate data, based on observation of the patient.
2. Protecting the patient from injury during a seizure.
3. Controlling seizure.
4. Rehabilitating and teaching the patient.

Providing accurate data based observation of the patient: Providing accurate data about the seizures, helps in accurate diagnosis. It requires a highly developed observational skills and an understanding of what to look for and how to record the observation.

The following points need to be considered when observing a seizure:

1. Were there any warning signs ?
2. Where did the seizure begin and how did it proceed ?
3. What type of movement was noted and what parts of the body involved ?
4. Were there any changes in the size of the pupils ?
5. Was there urinary or bowel incontinence ?
6. What was the duration of the entire attack and each phase?
7. Was the patient unconscious throughout the attack ?
8. What was the behavior of the patient after the attack ?
9. Did the patient sleep after the attack ?
10. Was there any postictal symptoms noticed ?

Care of the patient during seizure

1. If the patient experiences an aura prior to a convulsion have him lie down in order to prevent injury.

2. Provide for privacy by putting the bed curtains or screen (this protect the patient from embarrassment and curious on lookers).
3. Loosen tight clothings, if any.
4. Provide adequate ventilation.
5. Never leave the patient alone when he is having seizure.
6. Protect the head with a pad to prevent injury.
7. Push aside any furniture or things that may struck by the patient during the attack.
8. If the patient is in bed remove the pillow.
9. Remove spectacles if any to prevent injury.
10. Do not attempt to open jaws during the attack. No effort should be made to restrain the patient's extremities during the fit.
11. After the seizure keep the patient turned on his side to prevent aspiration.
12. Allow the patient to sleep after the seizure.
13. Re-orient the patient upon awakening, as amnesia may occur after the attack.

In the hospital, the epileptics should be put on seizure precautions; that means:

1. The side rails of the bed should be up and padded.
2. Suction set up and airway should be available at the bedside.
3. The bed is kept in a low position.

Controlling of seizures

Patients should be put on anticonvulsant drug. It can suppress seizures by either abolishing or reducing the amount of abnormal electrical activity in brain cells. Assess the effectiveness of the drug and observe for any signs of toxicity to the drug and report them immediately. Oral hygiene is stressed in preventing the complications of hypertrophy of the gums or gingivitis that may follow dilantin sodium therapy.

Patient education and rehabilitation

The following instructions to be given to the patient and family members:

1. To take tablets regularly, not missing even a single dose.
2. Patient may feel drowsy in the beginning. This should not lead to any change in drug dosage on his own.
3. Missing dose can result in a fit. Always keep stock of tablets ready for at least two weeks.

4. Never take the missed dose or doses cumulatively.
5. Keep them in a safe plastic container to avoid misuse of accidental use by other especially children.
6. Keep a small book and record the fits.
7. Regular follow-up is essential for adjustment of doses and assessment of any side effects.
8. Visit the doctor in the beginning once a fortnight, later once a month.
9. Till fits are fully under control do not work near fire, water, moving wheels, do not climb trees, and do not drive vehicles.
10. There is no food restrictions as part of treatment.
11. Continue all routine work, like going to school or work etc.
12. Patient should not be kept idle; he should be given a work to do and earn his livelihood, proper support and encouragement to be given so that he can live with pride and dignity.

SYNCOPE

Syncope is a brief loss of consciousness caused by sudden reduction of cerebral blood flow. Presyncope (fainting) refers to the situation in which there is reduction of cerebral blood flow and a sensation of impending loss of consciousness although the patient does not actually pass out.

Presyncope and syncope represent degrees of the same disorder and should be addressed as manifestation of the same underlying problem. Recovery from the syncope is usually complete once the patient collapses and the head is at the level of heart, consciousness is regained.

The physiologic causes of syncope fall under two categories:

- Decreased blood flow to the brain
- Altered state of blood to the brain, e.g. anemia and hypoxia.

The causes of syncope are:

1. Vasovagal syncope which results from vasodilatation of peripheral resistance vessels occurs in:
   - Physical injury
   - Strong emotions
   - Hot and crowded environment
   - Hyperventilation.
2. Postural hypotension (orthostatic) occurs in people with unstable or defective vasomotor reflexes from a variety of causes, e.g.
   - Prolonged bedrest

- Prolonged standing
- Drug side effects
- Peripheral nerve disfunction
- Hypovolemia.

3. Cardiac syncope—syncope occurs due to a sudden reduction in cardiac output usually because of dysrhythmia and structural cardiac defect.
4. Carotid sinus syncope—is due to an overly sensitive carotid sinus. Panting occurs when slight pressure is applied to the neck area where the carotid sinus is located, e.g. head turning while wearing a tight collar or even shaving over the region of carotid sinus.
5. Cerebral syncope occurs in case of
   - TIA
   - Hypertensive encephalopathy
   - Carotid, vertebral artery insufficiency
   - Various types of seizures.
6. Hematologic causes of syncope
   - Hypoglycemia
   - Anemia.
7. Pulmonary disorders—syncope may occur after paroxysms of coughing particulary in those suffering from cerebrovascular diseases and bronchitis, etc.
   - Cough syncope
   - Pulmonary hypertension
   - Pulmonary embolism.

Diagnosis is made by:
- History and examination
- Blood sugar estimation
- Radiograph of skull
- ECG
- EEG
- Reproducing syncopal attacks
- CT/MRI
- Cerebral angiography.

Management

- Rule out the medical causes of syncope
- Treat the cause of the disease.

Nursing Responsibility

- Patient should be made aware of his precipitating factors of syncope, its warning signs and take appropriate measures to prevent injury.
- Patients with uncontrolled syncopal attack should never be ambulated unassisted.
- Patient should be investigated thoroughly and proper cause should be identified and treatment given.
- Family should be educated about the illness, cause and treatment and their responsibility for the patient improvement.
- Till the diagnosis is made and treatment is given patient should be instructed
  1. Not to travel alone
  2. Not to ride the vehicle
  3. Not to swim
  4. Not to work near the fire
  5. Not to work near heavy machines.

12

Degenerative and Demyelinative Disorders of CNS

DEMENTIA

Definition

Dementia is an acquired, global impairment of intelligence, memory, and personality in the absence of impairment in the level of consciousness or it can be defined as global deterioration of acquired cognitive functions with a clear sensorium.

Dementia is not the same as normal aging. But about 65 percent of persons above the age of 65 suffer from dementia. Dementia occurs because of damage to brain tissue. It does not occur due to psychological factors. It may be associated with an underlying primary condition and may be reversible with prompt treatment of the primary problem.

Causes of Dementia

Dementia has many causes of which the most important are:

I. Degenerative disorders
   a. Alzheimer's disease
   b. Pick's disease
   c. Huntington's chorea
   d. Parkinson's disease
II. Intracranial space occupying lesions
   a. Tumor
   b. Subdural hematoma
III. Traumatic
   a. Severe head injury
   b. Repeated head injury in boxers and others

IV. Infection and related conditions
  a. Encephalitis
  b. Neurosyphilis
  c. Cerebral sarcoidosis
  d. HIV infection
V. Vascular
  a. Multiple cerebral vascular disease
  b. Occlusion of the carotid artery, cranial arteries
VI. Metabolic
  a. Sustained uremia
  b. Liver failure
  c. Remote effects of carcinoma and lymphoma
VII. Toxic
  a. Alcohol
  b. Poisoning with heavy metal (lead arsenic)
VIII. Anoxia
  a. Anemia
  b. Postanesthesia
  c. Chronic respiratory failure
IX. Vitamin deficiency
  a. Sustained lack of vitamin B_{12}
  b. Deficiency of folic acid, thiamin.

The major defects in dementia involve
- Memory impairment
- Psychosis
- Orientation impairment
- Neurological impairment
- Language impairment
- Catastrophic reactions
- Personality changes

Treatment and nursing management are same as Alzheimer's disease.

ALZHEIMER'S DISEASE

Alzheimer's disease is the most common cause of dementias. The disorder accounts for about half of all dementias. In Alzheimer's disease degenerative changes occur in the brain. The cause is not known. However, several chromosomal links have been identified. Females are more likely than males to be affected by this disease.

Definition

Alzheimer's disease is a chronic progressive degenerative disorder of the brain characterized by global impairment of cognitive functions.

Epidemiological findings suggest that 2 to 3 percent of elderly above 65 years may be suffering from AD in India. (Dr Indira Jai Prakash 1999).

Signs and Symptoms

The symptoms of AD can be best understood in the context of three stages of its manifestation.

Mild Alzheimer's Disease

- Difficulty in concentration
- Significant memory loss for recent events, for example some major events of the previous week are not recalled
- Disorientation to time
- Disorientation to place. Losing ones way in familiar places
- Difficulty in making decisions
- Lacking initiative and motivation
- Loss of interest in hobbies and activities
- Signs of depression and aggression.

Moderate and Moderately Severe Alzheimer's Disease

The deficits are large enough to prevent patients from surviving without assistance and they may require help in basic activities of daily living. At this stage they

- May become very forgetful especially for recent events
- May be unable to recall the names of people known to them
- Can no longer cook, keep the house clean or do shopping
- May become extremely dependent
- Need assistance with personal hygiene
- Has increasing difficulty with speech
- Many wander aimlessly and show behavioral abnormalities like sexual disinhibition, lack of concern and apathy towards self and others
- May experience delusions and hallucination.

The duration of this phase is approximately 4 years.

Severe Alzheimer's Disease

This stage is one of total dependence and inactivity. Memory disturbances are very serious and the physical side of the disease becomes more obvious.

The person may

- Have difficulty in eating
- Not recognize relatives, friends and family members
- Have difficulty in understanding and interpreting events
- Be unable to find the way around in the home
- Have difficulty in walking
- Bladder and bowel incontinence
- Inappropriate behavior in public
- Be confined to a wheelchair or bed.

Patient may survive in this stage for six years or longer. Pneumonia appears to be the most common proximate cause of deaths.

Diagnosis

Diagnosis is made by

- History
- Physical and mental status examination
- CT scan
- CSF analysis
- MRI.

Management of a Patient with Dementia

If the patient is suffering from treatable cause of dementia, therapy is directed toward treating the underlying disorder. There is no specific treatment for Alzheimer's disease. Some drugs have been marked to improve intellectual functions but these drugs produce little or no benefit.

The general treatment to a demented patient is to

1. provide supportive medical, nursing and psychosocial care,
2. emotional support for the patients and families, and
3. pharmacological treatment for specific symptoms.

Drug Treatment

There is no established specific drug treatment for dementia. Medication is used to alleviate certain symptoms.

Examples: Benzodiazepine for insomnia and anxiety
Antidepressants for depression
Antipsychotics for delusion and hallucination.

Nursing Management

1. *Assessment:* Careful and meticulous assessment of patient is very important before planning the nursing care.
   - Observe and analyze patient abilities to perform ADL, eating, bathing, dressing, etc.
   - Involve family members in planning and care.
2. *Maintaining peak physical health:* One of the most essential nursing action is to facilitate optional functioning by maintaining physical health.
   - Eye glasses for poor vision
   - Hearing aids for diminished hearing
   - Any other physical problem to be taken care of.
3. *Structuring the environment:* According to need and sensory level
   - Provide quiet and good lighting room
   - Provide orientation clues in the environment, like clocks, calenders, seasonal pictures, family photographs
   - Provide newspapers to know the current events
   - Use symbols to locate bathrooms rather than written signs
   - Remove any environmental hazards
   - Limit the number of family members, friends and visitors
   - Provide for frequent supervision.
4. *Promote communication and socialization:* As the patients will be disoriented, confused and will have problems in understanding. The caregiver should:
   - Approach very slowly.
   - Introduce at each interaction and explain what for she is there.
   - Verbal communication should be clear, concise and unhurried.
   - Questions that require 'yes' 'no' answers are best.
   - Watch for emotional and nonemotional cues for evidence of perception of communication.
   - Do not ask the patient to perform cognitive skills beyond his ability.

5. *Promoting independent functioning:*
   - Provide material for daily care available and accessible and encourage to do by themselves
   - Routine must be made simple and consistent
   - Enough time to be given to complete the task
   - Reinforce the activity to gain confidence.
6. *Providing physical need of the patient:*

   Nutrition
   - Provide food in small quantities at frequent intervals
   - Allow to eat at his own pace
   - Provide roughage and green leaf vegetables
   - Encourage fluids.

   Sleep
   - Control the patient's activity so that he will stay awake during day time.
   - Provide measures to facilitate sleep at night.

   Elimination
   - Any problems of elimination to be assessed and cared.
7. *Preserving family unit:* Care of a dementic patient is a full time and long-term care.
   - Patient's wife and relatives to be supported well
   - Education to family members regarding patient's condition and care to be explained
   - Family support groups and individual counselling may be organized
   - Linking them to some community-based services may be tremendous help for the family.

   Nursing care of older adults can be effectively achieved through a special ingredient. The special ingredient is respect, the courtesy, consideration and esteem due to each individual who has reached their age of life. This respect to be demonstrated in each nursing intervention.

PARKINSON'S DISEASE

Parkinson's disease is a chronic degenerative disorder of the basal ganglia of unknown etiology. The disease begins insidiously often unilaterally and progresses.

Etiology and Epidemiology

- Cause is unknown.
- It is a disease of elderly. Mean age of onset is 50 to 60 years.
- Men are affected slightly more often than women.

Pathology

The pathology is in basal ganglia.

The structures that compose the basal ganglia include the striatum, globus pallidum, subthalmic nucleus, *substantia nigra* and red nucleus.

In Parkinson's disease (because of degenerative changes) pigmented cells in the *substantia nigra* are lost and the dopamine stored in the cells is greatly reduced. The cell degeneration causes impairment of extrapyramidal tracts, semiautomatic functions and coordinated movements.

Signs and Symptoms

Symptoms develop very slowly. Years may pass before a diagnosis is made. The disease is progressive; eventually the patient may lose ability to perform ADL (activities of daily living) and may be confined to bed. The signs and symptoms include the following:

Major Manifestation

1. Muscle rigidity
2. Tremors
3. Bradykinesia
4. Postural instability/loss of postural reflexes.

Associated Manifestation

- Difficulty in fine motor functions, such as writing and eating
- Soft monotone voice
- Mask like face
- Visual defects
- General weakness and muscle fatigue
- Cognetive impairment
- Autonomic manifestation.

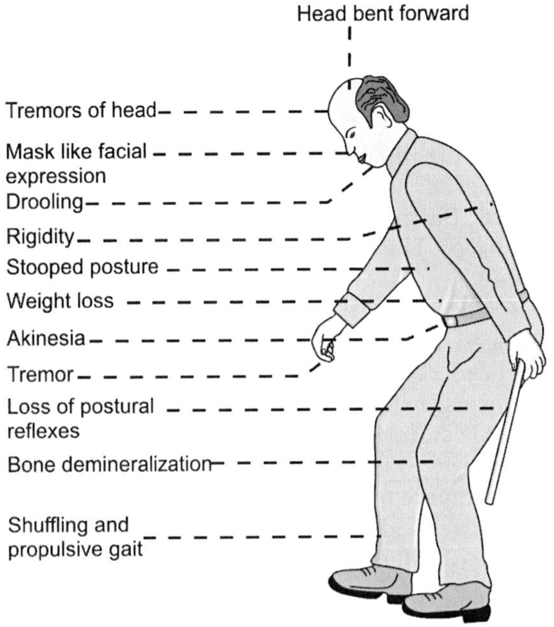

Fig. 12.1: Manifesting symptoms of Parkinson's disease

Major Manifestations (Fig. 12.1)

1. *Muscular rigidity:* The muscles become stiff and requires much effort to move.
2. *Tremors:* Tremors occur most often in the distal portions of extremities and especially in the hands. Also called 'Pill rolling' motion of the hands is characteristic of the disease. Other areas where tremors are seen include the foot, lip, tongue and jaw. Tremors are present when the hand is motionless and are absent during sleep.
3. *Bradykinesia:* The patient has difficulty initiating a movement. So moves slowly and performs ADL very slowly. Because of this slowness he has high risk for pneumonia, deep vein thrombosis, constipation and pressure sore.
4. *Postural disturbances:* The trunk of the body tend to stoop forward. The forearms are semiflexed and the fingers are flexed at the metacarpophalangeal joints. They usually walk in a stooped-over position with small, shuffling steps. The patient may fall forward or backward.

Associated Manifestation

1. *Difficulty with fine motor movements:* Difficulty with fine motor control will be present. Handwriting becomes progressively smaller and more difficult to read.
   Clumsiness and difficulty will be seen in his ADL activities, such as buttoning of clothing is evident.
2. *Visual defects:* Blurred vision is common.
3. *Monotonic voice:* The voice gradually becomes soft monotonic and muffled.
4. *Mask like face:* The face is expressionless and the eyes stare straight ahead. Blinking is less frequent than normal. No smile will be noticed.
5. *General weakness and muscle fatigue:* Patient becomes tired very easily. Muscle cramps of the legs, neck and trunk are common.
6. *Cognitive changes:* Decline in thinking capacity, memory deficits and depression are more common.
7. *Other autonomic manifestations:*
   - Drooling of saliva
   - Seborrhea
   - Dysphasia
   - Excessive perspiration
   - Constipation
   - Orthostatic hypotension
   - Urinary hesitation.

Diagnosis

Diagnosis is made by
1. History and physical examination
2. Lumbar puncture
3. EEG
4. CT
5. MRI
6. PETT (positron emission transaxial tomography).

Medical Management

There is no treatment to arrest the degeneration of basal ganglia. But drugs relieves many symptoms of parkinsonism.
1. Levadopa or syndopa is the main drug used. It converts to dopamine in the basal ganglia, thereby relieves the symptoms of rigidity and bradykinesia.

It is given 100 to 200 mg per day, according to the patients in 2 doses. In the night usually the dosage is avoided as the symptoms are less during sleep.

2. Anticholinergic drugs used in conjuction with L. dopa to relieve tremors. Trihexy phenidyl (artane 2 mg tds is given).
3. Amantadine hydrochloride (symmetrel) 100 to 300 mg per day divided 2 to 3 times a day. It is a rapid acting drug. Improves all symptoms.
4. Selegiline IV (Neuroprotective agent) 5 to 10 mg per day divided, two times a day.

Surgical Treatment

Severe Parkinson disease requires stereotactic surgery where parts of the basal ganglia are destroyed. The purpose of the surgery is to reduce tremors and rigidity.

Nursing Care of Parkinson Disease

Parkinson disease is a slow progressive disease where the patient has impaired physical mobility, muscle rigidity with weakness, and autonomic disturbances. Nursing care consists of:

A. *Improving mobility and functioning:*
- Provide for range of motion exercises 4 times a day.
- Emphasize the importance of a daily exercise program (walk, swim, garden work) to maintain joint mobility.
- Advise the patient to do stretching exercises (stretch -hold-relax) to loosen the joint structures.
- Advise the patient to have frequent rest periods.
- Encourage to take warm baths, massage and passive and active exercises.
- Evaluate the effectiveness of the drug program and adjust as necessary:

B. *Gaining independence in self care:*
1. Teach the patient how to turn and get out of bed.
   a. Bend the knees and turn upper half of body, the lower half of the body will follow.
   b. To get out of bed, turn on side and then place feet over the edge of bed and push up with the arm.
2. Use assistive devices to help in bathing and grooming, e.g. long-handled bath brush, soap or rope, button aids, etc.

C. *Preventing injury:*
- Remove environmental objects that could cause falls.
- Provide assistive devices to support mobility.
- Secure a knotted rope to foot of bed to allow patient to pull himself to a sitting position.
- Refer to physiotherapist for postural and gait training.

D. *Improving nutritional status:*
- Teach the patient how to eat with his disability.
- Encourage to make conscious effort to chew and to chew first on one side and then the other.
- Control the build up of saliva by holding head in an upright position and making a conscious effort to swallow.
- Have patient/family keep a weekly weight chart.
- Arrange for supplementary feedings to augment caloric intake.

E. *Maximizing residual communication ability:*
- Accept the patient's attempts to communicate.
- Speech therapy may be given for patient with verbal deficit.
- For writing difficulty, develop an alternative method of communication.
- Remind patient of the following.
  a. Take a deep breath before speaking.
  b. speak in short sentence.
  c. Practice breathing exercise regularly.
- Exercise facial muscle (smile, frown grimace) for facial mobility.
- Advice the patient to practice reading aloud in front of a mirror to improve speech.

F. *Providing psychological support and social interaction:*
- Develop a trusting relationship and adopt positive attitude towards others
- Allow the patient to express his/her feelings of frustration, anger, depression, guilt, etc.
- Be supportive and give positive reinforcement for his/her achievements in ADL.

G. *Patient/Family teaching:*
- Patient and family to be taught about the disease condition, treatment, and care of patient, etc.
- They can be encouraged to participate in supportive group if available.

MULTIPLE SCLEROSIS (MS)

Nerve cell is covered by a sheath called myelin sheath composed of a white, lipid substance that acts as an insulator for the conduction of impulses. The destruction of myelin sheath of nerve cell causes some diseases in CNS. Diseases in which the normal myelin is disrupted are considered demyelinating diseases.

Definition

Multiple sclerosis (MS) or disseminated sclerosis is a chronic, progressive, degenerative disease that affects the myelin sheath and conduction pathways of the central nervous system (CNS). The illness is characterized by periods of remission and exacerbation. Early in the disease, the periods between the exacerbations will be longer than at late stages. As the illness progresses, the period of exacerbations are closer together with the severity and duration of each exacerbation increasing.

Etiology and Epidemiology

The etiology of MS is unknown. Theories of causation include:
1. Viral infection
2. Autoimmune response
3. Hereditary.

Many studies have ascertained that
- Incidence is more between the age group of 20 to 40 years. Twenty percent patients experience their first symptom in their 40s and 50s.
- Women are more affected than men—2:1.
- More prevalent in the colder northern latitudes.
- Relatives of patients are at greater risk than general population.

Pathophysiology

The name 'Multiple Sclerosis' is derived from the multiplicity of lesions with sclerotic appearance on cut section of myelin sheaths.

The disease affects the white matter of the brain and spinal cord by causing scattered, demyelinated lesions of the long conduction pathways of the CNS. The destruction of myelin sheath surrounding the axons leaves patches of sclerotic tissue. Nerve fibers degenerate so that the disabilities increases and becomes permanent. Upon autopsy, multiple sclerotic plaques are scattered throughout white matter of the brain and spinal cord. The neurological deficits are apparent during the periods of exacerbation and can completely disappear during remission. Remission occurs due to healing of the demyelinated area by sclerotic tissue. Eventually symptoms becomes permanent because of nerve fiber degeneration.

Signs and Symptoms

The signs and symptoms of MS are varied and may be vague. Initial symptoms can occur alone or in any combination. They are:

1. *Sensory symptoms*
   - Numbness and tingling the face or involved extremities
   - Anesthesia/paresthesia
   - Decreased propriception (sense of position) and sense of temperature, objective sensory loss (position vibration and shape)
   - Pain is uncommon except flexor spasm
   - Lhermittes sign—electric shock or shock like sensation that extends down the arm, back or lower trunk upon flexor of neck. This is due to bukling effect of the dorsal roots from sclerotic plaques.
2. *Motor symptoms*
   - Weakness in the lower extremities (paresis)
   - Start with one limb and later both limbs will be involved, dragging of foot may be present
   - Spasticity of limbs interferes ambulation and ADL
   - Bladder and bowel dysfunction—incontinence or retention
   - Uhthoff's sign—decline in motor function after exposure to a hot bath is a diagnostic test of MS.
3. *Cerebellar function*
   - Ataxia
   - Loss of balance and coordination
   - Intentional tremor—a tremor occurring when a voluntary act is initiated
     The finer the movement the greater the tremor
   - Speech disturbance, dysarthria, dystonia, scanning speech. Scanning of speech is defined as speech that is slow and measured with pause between syllables.

4. *Other symptoms*
   - Fatigue
   - Opticneuritis causing visual clouding and visual field deficits and pain, diplopia and nystagmus
   - Impotence and sexual dysfunction
   - Neurobehavioral problems such as depression or euphoria.

Precipitating Factors

Events that may precipitate relapses are:
- Fatigue
- Infection
- Exertion
- Emotional stress
- Cold
- Humid or hot weather
- Hot baths
- Fever
- Menstruation, etc.

Course of Illness

The course of multiple sclerosis is unpredictable. The MS is classified according to the clinical course of the condition. They are as follows:

1. *Relapse/remitting disease:* In this type, the relapse occur within 1 to 2 weeks of remission and return gradually to baseline over a period of 4 to 8 weeks. Almost 65 percent of the cases do occur in this way.
2. *Relapsing/progressing:* In this type, the patient never comes to baseline but left with some significant residual disability.
3. *Chronic progressive type:* In this type, the onset is more insidious and the course if progressive without remission.
4. *Stable MS:* In this type, the patient may go without any active clinical symptoms for a year or more. But when the clinical symptoms occur there will be deficits within 3 months which will be permanent.

Prognosis is impossible to predict. Some will live a normal life. Other patients may die from infections of urinary and respiratory system. Some others may live with deficits.

Diagnosis

Diagnosis to done by
1. History and physical examination
2. MRI
3. Evoked potential
4. CSF
5. PET.

Treatment

Treatment of MS is symptomatic and supportive. The supportive therapy can be with drugs and physiotherapy. There is no specific treatment.

Drugs are:
1. Methyl prednisolone is given in the acute stage as 1 gm IV for 5 days. (infusion). Later depending upon clinical course oral prednisolone is given.
2. Tab baclofen and diazepam may be added to control spasticity.

Physiotherapy

The goal of the physiotherapy is to see the patient as independent as possible for as long as possible. Methods and devices can be employed to allow for ambulation, self-feeding, dressing and other ADL.

Nursing Management

Nursing management consists of
1. Improve the functioning ability of the patient
   a. Strengthen muscles and prevent and treat muscle spasticity
      - Make the patient to do muscle stretching exercises daily to minimize spasticity, joint contractures and tightening and shortening of certain muscle groups.
      - Teach the patient's family passive exercises and range of motion exercises for patients with severe spasticity.
      - Maintain proper body alignment when in and out of bed.
      - Provide supportive shoes and devices like splints, slings or pillows to support the affected extremities.

   b. Advise the patient to avoid muscle fatigue. Stop physical activity just short of fatigue and take frequent, short rest periods, preferably lying down.

c. Encourage the patient to sleep prone at intervals to minimize flexor spasms at knees and hips.
d. Encourage to participate in walking exercises.
e. Utilise braces, canes, crutches, walker, when necessary to keep the patient ambulatory.

2. Compensate for sensory impairment: Patients will have sensory and perceptual alteration (visual, auditory, kinesthetic and tactile).
   a. Monitor the function of all senses.
   b. Make the environment safe.
   c. For kinesthetic and tactile alterations.
      - Talk to the patient while giving care and tell him what you are doing.
      - Provide tactile stimulation to the affected part.
      - Tell the patient to protect affected parts around cold or heat.
   d. For visual alteration
      - Arrange personal articles and necessary items on unaffected side.
      - Approach the patient from the unaffected side.
      - Use eye patch, to block visual impulses of one eye when the patient has diplopia.
3. Conserve energy to relieve fatigue
   - Help the patient to understand that fatigue is an integral part of MS and not to feel guilty
   - Plan ahead, list priorities,
   - Plan time for rest and pace self throughout day.
   - Avoid overheating (hot baths), over exertion and infection.
   - Develop a lifestyle promoting wellness, use balanced diet. Low in fat, balance rest and exercise and avoid anything that aggravate symptoms.
4. Prevent injury
   - Assist the patient to overcome effects of incoordination.
   - Teach the patient to walk with feet wider apart—to widen his base of support and increase his walking stability.
   - Inform the patient to avoid abrupt change in position to be careful in turning, sitting and standing.
   - Use weighted bracelets, wrist-cuffs to help overcome in coordination of upper extremities.

5. Assist in maintaining personal hygiene
   - Identify factors that limit performance of ADL.
   - Provide for basic care that the patient cannot provide for self and demonstrate the use of assistive devices to maintain his/her personal hygiene.
6. Establish bladder control
   - Monitor the frequency and amount of urine voided.
   - Ascertain the type of bladder problem present and take necessary action.
   - Emphasise that bacterial urinary tract infection is common in MS neurologic dysfunction increases when fever is present. Report immediately.
7. Achieve bowel control
   - Monitor bowel movement for frequency and consistency.
   - Teach appropriate techniques and methods to have regular bowel movement.
8. Strive toward increased independence in self care activities.
   - Make occupational therapy referral for evaluation of structural arrangement of work place and home.
   - Secure proper wheelchair with features that will maximize mobility.
   - Use assistive and modified self help devices for toilet facilities, bathing facilities and self care facilities.
9. Attain/maintain skin integrity
   - Take necessary precautions to prevent pressure sores.
10. Adapt to sexual dysfunction
    - Discuss the possibility of sexual dysfunction with the patient.
    - Establish whether dysfunction is present.
    - Encourage open communication between partners.
    - Make appropriate referrals.
11. Provide necessary psychological support and help to maintain self concept
    - Allow the patient to express feelings/indicate your understanding and acceptance.
    - Correct misconceptions.
    - Be supportive, help the patient to develop his strategies to deal with change.
    - Identify support groups (MS society) in the community and refer the patient.

12. Maintain family integrity:
    - See that care givers of MS patients maintain their health and social life.
    - Help the family to get community resources for financial help and other support.

Discharge Planning/Patient Education

- Patient and family should be educated about the illness, course, cause, treatment and outcome and care of patient with MS.
- Should be educated about the relapse and necessary care to prevent relapse of MS.

RETROBULBAR NEURITIS (OPTIC NEURITIS)

The condition is due to a patch of demyelination developing in one optic nerve. Most commonly, it is an early stage of multiple sclerosis or it may occur in isolation. Later on the other nerve may be affected and some times both at once.

Signs and Symptoms

- Pain in the eye
- Blurring of vision, progressing to complete loss of vision
- Papillitis and optic atrophy can be seen through ophthalmoscope.

Course

Functional vision is restored within 2 weeks in 25 percent of patients and within 2 months in another 50 percent of patients but require 1 year for the remaining patients. Recurrence occurs in approximately 10 to 15 percent of patients within first year.

Treatment

IV methyl prednisolone 250 mg every 6 hours for 3 days followed by oral prednisolone 1 mg/kg per day for 11 days, speeds the recovery of visual loss in severe optic neuritis.

Nursing Care

- Proper explanation about the disease condition and necessary psychological support to be given.

MOTOR NEURON DISEASE

The term motor neuron disease (MND) encompasses a spectrum of disease, characterized by degeneration of upper and/or lower motor neurons in the brain, spinal cord or both.

In some MNDs only upper motor neurons (UMNs) are affected, e.g. progressive pseudobulbar palsy and hereditary spastic paraplegia.

In some only the lower motor neurons (LMNSs) are affected, e.g.

- Progressive bulbar palsy
- Progressive muscular atrophy
- Spinal muscular atrophy

The combination of UMN and LMN involvement is called amyotrophic lateral sclerosis.

AMYOTROPHIC LATERAL SCLEROSIS (ALS)

It is a rapidly progressing, fatal, degenerative disease of the upper and lower motor neurons. It is characterized by destruction of motor neurons in the brainstem, and in the anterior gray horns of the spinal cord, along with degeneration of pyramidal tracts. Resulting in wasting of the muscles of the body. If the lower motor neurons are involved weakness, wasting (atrophy) and fasciculations will be present. If upper motor neurons are involved hyperreflexes and spasticity, sensory changes are not a part of the disease.

Causes and Incidence

- Cause of ALS is unknown
- Slow virus is probable cause
- Genetic components in some families may be present
- Men are more affected than women (3 times more).

Pathophysiology

There are marked degenerative changes in the following structure:

1. Anterior horn cells of the spinal cord.
2. Motor nuclei of the brainstem (especially cranial nerves of VII facial and XII hypoglossal).
3. Corticospinal tract, beta cells and precentral cells of the frontal cortex.

Upper motor neuron involvement results in spasticity and weakness of muscles, whereas lower motor neuron involvement causes flaccidity, paralysis and muscle atrophy. Sensory functions, intellectual ability, vision and hearing are not affected.

Signs and Symptoms

- Weakness and wasting atrophy of muscles. The muscles most commonly affected are the intrinsic muscles of the hand as evident by clumsiness. Later on shoulder and upper arm muscles and in the last lower limbs are affected. Patient will feel heavy and easily fatigued of muscles.
- Muscle spasticity and hyper-reflexes.
- Fasciculations of muscle causes twitching.
- When brainstem is involved, atrophy of tongue will be present causing dysarthria. The tongue will have fasciculation.
- Muscle of speech, chewing and swallowing may be affected leading to dysphagia.
- Dyspnea (when respiratory muscles are involved).
- Fatigue.
- Weakness of all the limbs.

Diagnosis

- EMG (electromyogram)
- CPK (creatine phosphokinase)
- Myelogram.

Treatment

ALS is incurable. But the new treatment may slow the progress of the disease. Riluzole 50 mg PO bd (glutamate antagonist) delays the progress of the disease so that tracheostomy is postponed.

Many treatments are under trial, which include cyclophosphamide.

Patients are managed with:

- Physiotherapy
- Occupational therapy
- Speech therapy
- Periodic assessment of respiratory function and monitoring
- Gastrostomy tube feeding

- Ongoing counseling
- Drug therapy for various problems like spasticity, cramps, sialorrhea.

Course of Illness

It is a rapidly growing progressing disease, in which 50 percent of the victims are dead three years after onset.

Nursing Management

No treatment can currently arrest ALS. The nurses' role is:

1. Assisting the patient to be as independent and comfortable as possible.
2. Providing emotional and psychological support for the patient and family.
3. Giving education about the disease condition and treatment and outcome of the disease to the patient and family.
4. Limiting the development of complications.
5. Assisting in special therapeutic regimes, such as physical therapy, speech therapy and occupational therapy.
6. Providing spiritual support.
7. Helping the patient to make decisions about advance directives, hospice care and getting his or her affairs in order.
8. Preparing for death, reassurance of a comfortable death.
9. Providing information about support groups.

As a whole the nurses' role in caring motor neuron disease is symptoms oriented and psychological support to patient and the family members.

GUILLAIN-BARRÉ SYNDROME (POLYRADICULONEURITIS)

Guillain-Barré syndrome is an acute inflammatory demyelinating polyneuropathy of the peripheral nerves characterized by a rapid onset of weakness and often paralysis of extremities and respiratory muscles.

Incidence

1.7% per 100,000.

Causes

- The etiology is unknown

- Believed to be an autoimmune response to viral infection
- There may be history of acute infection such as upper respiratory infection, viral pneumonia or GI infection or patient receiving a vaccination which trigger to self-off autoimmune response to damage the peripheral nerves.

Pathology

This disease primarily affects the motor components of peripheral nerves. There will be destruction of the myelin sheath surrounding cranial and spinal nerves, edema and inflammation takes place. The demyelination of axon causes in loss of saltatory conduction and the axonal injury leads to reduction in amplitude of muscle potential and signals a poorer recovery. The demyelinization begins in the distal nerves and ascends symmetrically. The demyelination is patchy and the remyelination process occurs very slowly.

Clinical Manifestation

1. Symmetrical motor weakness beginning in the legs and the progressing to the trunk and arms.
2. Respiratory failure.
3. Facial (VII) glossopharyngeal (IX), vagus (X), spinal accessory (XI), and hypoglossal (XII) nerves may be affected causing facial paralysis, difficulty in chewing, swallowing, drinking and talking.
4. Paresthesia—tingling, numbness, abnormal sensation, vibrations and crawling sensations.
5. Autonomic dysfunction—tachycardia, blood pressure changes, bladder dysfunction.
6. Pain which is aching or cramping worst at night, interferes with sleep.

   GBS does not affect the level of consciousness cognitive function or papillary changes.

Diagnosis

1. Clinical history
2. CSF
3. EMG studies.

Medical Management

The usual line of management is either IVIG (intravenous immunoglobulin) as 400 mg/kg x 5 days or plasmapheresis (large/small) volume and supportive treatment.

Complications of the Disease

- Respiratory failure
- Cardiac arrhythmia
- Complications of paralysis—pressure sores and contractures
- Urinary retention
- Psychological problems (depression, fear, etc.)

Course of the Disease

There are three stages of acute GBS

1. *Acute onset:* Begins with the onset of first symptom and ends when no further symptoms, usually 1 to 3 weeks.
2. *Plateu period:* Lasts for several days to 2 weeks.
3. *Recovery period:* Period of remyelination and axonal regeneration.

In some patients sustained secondary axonal injury takes two years for maximal improvement with permanent deficits.

Nursing Management

When the signs and symptoms of GBS develop the chief concern is respiratory insufficiency because of neuromuscular weakness. Many patient require intubation and ventilatory support. Nursing intervention is directed towards maintaining adequate respiration, maintaining patent airway, preventing pulmonary infection and preventing complications of immobility.

As patients are conscious, have breathing problems and put on ventilators they will be very fearful and have fear of dying. They need continued support and reinforcement of the fact that the outcome is optimistic.

The nursing care consists of

a. Maintaining breathing when rapidly ascending paralysis develops.

- Anticipate the risk of respiratory failure, observe progression of patients weakness and paralysis.
- Monitor for pulse rate of over 120 beats/minutes or under 70 beats/minute, evaluate respiratory rate >30 breaths/minute.
- Watch for breathlessness while talking, shallow and irregular breathing, increasing pulse rate and change in respiratory pattern.
- Administer oxygen as needed.
- Prepare patient for intubation and ventilatory support when signs of deteriorating respiratory function are noted.
- Talk to the patient and explain what is being done to alleviate patients anxiety.
- When on ventilator ensure safe use within the parameter set for the ventilation.

b. Maintaining effective airway clearance as patient has weakness of cough reflex and respiratory muscle.
  - Position the patient on the side to facilitate the draining from airway, elevate the head end to 30° angle.
  - Suction the airway to maintain potency.
  - Administer chest physiotherapy every 2 to 4 hours.
  - If tracheostomy is present, provide the tracheostomy every 4-hourly.

c. Compensating for loss of mobility
  - Position the patient correctly to avoid further damage to susceptible peripheral nerves, pressure sores and contracture.
  - Provide range of motion exercises.
  - Elevate lower leg (35–40 degree) periodically to relieve edema.
  - Promote venous return by applying thigh high elastic stockings.

d. Coping with communication loss
  - Teach how to communicate within physical limitation.
  - Have some type of call or alarm system.
  - Maintain eye contact while speaking to the patient.
  - Use diversional therapy (family visits, cassette, tapes, music).

e. Maintaining nutrition
  - Ausculate lower abdomen for bowel sounds.
  - Use nasogastric tube for feeding.

- Reassure that this is short-term management.
- Be prepared to resume oral feedings when pharyngeal muscles are strong enough to prevent aspiration.

f. Maintain bladder and bowel movement
- Establish bladder retaining program (intermittent catheterization) as per the physician protocol.
- Monitor intake output chart.
- Maintain bowel program.

g. Provide measures to reduce pain due to peripheral nerve injury
- Observe the character and pattern of pain.
- Enhance comfort through positioning.
- Teach imagery and relaxation technique.
- Administer analgesic as ordered.

h. Relieving fear
- Offer continuing reassurance, explanation and high level care as the patient is alert, anxious and has vision and hearing.
- Clarify misconceptions that contribute to fear.
- Reassure him by pointing out gains being made. Chart improvements as this allows patients to assess progress.

i. Establish effective sleeping pattern.

j. Discharge planning and patient education
- Make them to realize that convalescence may be lengthy and that recovery may taken 3 months to 2 years.
- Develop a teaching plan to help the patient and family members about the illness.
- Encourage breathing exercises to redevelop well-coordinated pattern of respiration.
- Avoid over fatigue.
- Avoid excessive weight gain.
- Teach the patient to check feet for injuries as minor trauma may go unnoticed because of sensory impairment.
- Contact Guillain-Barré syndrome support group for group support.

(Plasmapheresis and its nursing management is discussed in other chapter of this book)

13

Congenital Abnormalities of Nervous System

As it happens in any other part of the human body, nervous system also can have abnormalities during its developmental stage and will be noticed after the child is born. Few major and more common conditions and their management will be discussed in this chapter.

HYDROCEPHALUS

It is defined as the dilatation of ventricles of the brain because of the increased accumulation of cerebrospinal fluid. It means there is an imbalance between the production and absorption of CSF in the individual or it can be an obstruction in the pathway of CSF. Congenital hydrocephalus can be classified as,

a. Communicating
b. Noncommunicating

Communicating: No obstruction in the pathway of CSF circulation. But there is an increase in CSF production or the absorption is less.

Noncommunicating: It means the production and absorption of CSF is balanced but there is an obstruction in the pathway of CSF circulation.

Etiology

1. Increased production of CSF due to the infection of chorionic villi of ventricles of brain.
2. Decrease in the rate of absorption of CSF due to subdural hematoma/infection.
3. Obstruction in the pathway of CSF due to
   a. Stenosis
   b. Tumors

c. Spina bifida
d. Meningocele
e. Meningomyelocele.

Signs and Symptoms

They depend upon the age of the child whether cranial sutures closed or not.

Infants

a. Increase in size of the head.
b. Delayed closure of anterior fontanelle. Fontanelle may become tense and elevated above the surface of the skull.
c. Signs of increased ICP
   - Vomiting, restlessness, irritability, high pitched and shrill cry.
   - Alteration in vital signs, pupillary changes, seizures, lethargy, stupor.
d. Alteration of muscle tone of the extremities.
e. Later physical changes:
   - Forehead becomes prominent
   - Scalp appears shiny with prominent scalp vein
   - Eyebrows and eyelids may be drawn downward exposing the sclera above the iris
   - Infant cannot gaze upward causing "sunset eyes"
   - Strabismus, nystagmus and optic atrophy may occur
   - Infant has difficulty in holding head up
   - Later may experience physical and mental developmental delay.

In older children who have closed suture

Increased ICP with

1. Headache
2. Vomiting
3. Lethargy, fatigue, apathy
4. Personality changes
5. Separation of cranial sutures
6. Double visison, sudden appearance of internal strabismus, pupillary changes.
7. Alteration in vital sign as in infants, stupor
8. Coma

Diagnosis

1. Physical examination
2. Percussion of infant's skull may produce a typical 'cracked' pot sound (Macewen's sign)
3. Ophthalmoscopy
4. CT scan
5. X-ray.

Treatment

1. Surgery and removal of the obstruction.
2. Intracranial shunt in selected cases of noncommunicating hydrocephalis to divert the fluid from the obstructed segment to the subarachnoid space beyond the block.
3. Extracranial shunt—Divert from the ventricular system into extracranial compartment frequently into peritoneum or right atrium.
4. If the cause is infection appropriate drugs are given.

Common Extracranial Shunt

1. Ventriculoperitoneal shunt (V.P. shunt)
   - From the lateral ventricle or the subarachnoid space to the peritoneal cavity.
2. Ventriculoatrial shunt (V.A. shunt)
   - A tube is passed from the dilated ventricle through a burrhole in the parietal region of the skull to right atrium of heart.

Complications

- Need for shunt revision frequently occurs because of occlusion, infection, malfunction.
- Shunt revision may be necessary because of the growth of the child, where the length of the tube becomes small for the child.

Prognosis

1. Depends upon early diagnosis and prompt therapy
2. Success of surgical intervention

Nursing Management

1. *Measure head*
   Occipitofrontal circumference be measured daily at same time.
2. *Observe for evidence of increased ICP*
   a. Change in LOC
   b. Change in vital sign
      i. Increased systolic pressure
      ii. Decreased pulse rate
      iii. Decreased and irregular respiratory rate
   c. Vomiting
   d. Pupillary changes.
3. *Note especially these changes in appearance*
   - Increased head size/prominent forehead
   - Full bulging fontanelle
   - Sunset eyes
   - Opisthotonic positioning (occurs with brainstem herniation).
4. *Provide adequate nutrition*
   - Offer small frequent feeding
   - Hold the infant in a semisitting position with head well supported
   - Allow ample time for bubbling
   - Place the child on his side with his head elevated after feeding.
5. *Assist in diagnostic procedures*
   - Explain the procedure to parents
   - Administer prescribed medication
   - Observe carefully.
6. *Provide supportive nursing care*
   - Prevent pressure sore and development of contractures
   - Alternative pressure mattres or a sponge rubber mattres
   - Keep the scalp clean and dry
   - Change position 2nd hrly (head and body turn at sametime) A pillow at the side to support head and shoulder
   - Provide meticulous skin care
   - Provide range of motion exercises.

   Eye care
   - If the child is not closing the eyes, the eyes should be moistered.

   Provide for the child's emotional need for love and affection.
   - Hold and cuddle
   - Play with the child.

Provide emotional support to the parents
- Provide appropriate informations
- Correct misconceptions.

Postoperative Nursing Care

1. Provide immediate supportive nursing care:
   - Monitor the child's TPRBP pupillary changes—every 15 minutes until fully in reactive, then monitor for 1 to 2 hours.
   - Avoid hypothermia or hyperthermia
   - Aspirate whenever is necessary
   - Turn the child every 2 hours.
2. Allow for optimal drainage of cerebrospinal fluid.
   - Pump the shunt and position the child as directed.
   - If pumping is prescribed carefully compress the valve at specified number of times.
3. Prevent the development of pressure sores.
   - Avoid positioning the child on the area of the valve.
4. Maintain fluid and electrolyte balance
5. Observe for signs of complications
   - Increased ICP
   - Dehydration
   - Infections
   - Excessive drainage of fluid from the cranial cavity.
6. Provide continued emotional support.
7. Initiate appropriate referrals.

Advice on Discharge

- Teach the parents to watch for any signs of increased ICP.
- Teach them the initial care to be done in case of any increased ICP.
- Advice them to come immediately for further management like change of tube, reshunt, etc.
- Give them the guidances to prevent congenital abnormalities for the next pregnancy like
  - Avoid certain drugs during pregnancy.
  - Avoid radiation during early pregnancy.
  - Avoid infection during early pregnancy.
  - Avoid any type of fall, accidents during early pregnancy, if occurs report to the physician.

SPINA BIFIDA

It is a malformation of the spine in which the posterior position of the laminae of the vertebrae fails to close.

Many types are there, but three common types are as follows:

1. *Spina bifida occulta:* defect is only in the vertebrae.
2. *Meningocele:* in which the meninges protrude through the opening in the spinal canal forming cyst, filled with CSF and covered with skin.
3. *Meningomyelocele (Myelomeningocele):* Both spinal cord and cord membranes protrude through the defect in the laminae of the spinal canal. They are covered with thin membrane.

Etiology

1. Unknown—Genetic predisposition
2. Arrest in during 4 to 6th week of embryogenesis.

Incidence

- Geographical distribution
- Most common developmental defects of CNS
- May have associated congenital anomalies
- Women who have spina bifida and parents who have one affected child have an increased risk of producing children with neural tube defects.

Spina Bifida Occulta

- Most common type—25 percent of normal children have.
- Defect may vary for a thin slit separating one lamina from the spinous process to a complete absence of the spines and laminae.
- Most patients have no symptoms. There may be a dimple in the skin or growth of hair.
- As they do not give symptoms, they are diagnosed casually when the spine is X-rayed for any other reasons.

MENINGOCELE

It is a condition where the meninges are protruded congenitally through the spina bifida with CSF usually.

Signs and Symptoms

1. A visible sacular protrution in the back which may not be covered by the skin.
2. Decreased motor and sensory control below of the level of lesion.
3. Associated problems like talepes.
4. Associated neurological problems like Arnold-Chiari malformation.
5. Hydrocephalus, etc.
6. Urological problems.
7. Physical and mental disability is common.

Management

Management is surgical removal of meninges and closure of spina bifida if indicated and possible, that is

1. The child should have the stamina to withstand the surgery and anesthesia.
2. The lesion should be small enough to do the surgery to have improvement in symptoms.
3. Child should have only manageable problems associated with meningocele.

Nursing Management

1. Keep the child on abdomen to prevent rupture of the meningocele
2. Keep the bulge moist with vascline gauge
3. Transfer the child to a pediatrician or neurosurgeon as early as possible
4. Give emotional support to the parents.

MENINGOMYELOCELE

This is a congenital condition in which the meninges along with part of spinal cord is protruded through the spina bifida.

Signs and Symptoms

1. Sacular protrution in CSF seen at the back.
   Common sites are sacral and rarely cervical.

2. Decreased muscular tone of the limbs.
3. Associated congenital problems in lower limbs as talepes.
4. Hydrocephalus and associated symptoms.

Clinical Problems

A. Neurologic problems
   1. Arnold-Chiari malformation
      - Associated malformation involving brainstem and cerebellum
      - Hydrocephalus
   2. Loss of motor control and sensation below the level of the lesion.

B. Mobility and orthopedic problems
   1. Contractures may occur in the ankles, knees and hips
   2. Club feet are common (due to parplegic feet in the uterus)
   3. Scoliosis is common in later years
   4. Ambulation and ability to upright are possible, by using various types of bracing and equipment.

C. Urological problem
   - Unable to empty urine leading to urinary infections because of constant retention
   - Incontinence

D. Bowel problem
   - Fecal incontinence or constipation

E. Skin problems

F. Dietary problems—becomes overweight due to inactivity or underweight due to poor intake.

G. Developmental problems
   - Low intelligence
   - Handicaps.

Diagnosis

1. Physical examination
2. CT scan if necessary.

Management

Surgical removal of the sac and put back the meninges along with the spinal tissue through the spina bifida. This is done if the child is fit to undergo the surgery.

Contraindications for surgery are

- Physical unfitness of the child to withstand anesthesia and surgery.
- Extensive associated problems where the surgery may not help much.
- Local infections.

Nursing Management

- Prevention of infection.
- Prevention of break of the sac.
- Prevention of nutritional and fluid deficiency.
- Prevention of respiratory problems as the child is put on abdomen most of the time to prevent rupture of the sac.
- Keep the sac almost moist, do not allow it to dry.
- Prevent ulcers and sores of any prominent part of the body which rubs with the bed, as the child is kept on abdomen and childs muscle tone is inadequate.
- Emotional support to the parents and to the relatives should be continuous.
- Advice on discharge should include the counselling of the future pregnancy and childbirth.

Prevention

1. Prenatal detection through amniocentesis and measurement of alpha fetoprotein (risk group), where termination of pregnancy is possible.

Nursing Care in Labor Room

1. Children born with visible meningocele or meningomyelocele should be kept where absolute sterile nursing care can be given.
2. Special care is given to position the child to prevent the rupture of the sac.
3. The sac is prevented from getting touched with any infected materials.
4. Refer the child to the neurosurgeons as early as possible.

Defective Head Growth

Three major problems are found.

1. *Microcephaly:* This is underdevelopment of head. True microcephaly is a recessive inherited disorder where mature brain weighs less than 1000 gm. Other features associated are small fontanels, flat occipit, pointed vertex, receding forehead, stunted growth, retardation of speech, retardation of cognitive mental capacities.
   Treatment: Is rehabilitation with holistic approach for maximum development.
2. *Craniostenosis:* It is a group of condition where in two or more cranial bones unite prematurely, so that the cranial appearance is distorted. Brain may be normal but the symptoms are related to inadequacy of cranial capacity. Distortion of head and face depends upon which sutures are involved.
   Management: Is individualized since children are diagnosed at various points and thus have varying problems in relation to development. Sometimes surgical interventions also advised.
3. *Macrocephaly:* It is a problem related to embryonic growth or progressive disease process that results in abnormal cellular and structural changes in brain tissue. This abnormal growth may be a result of a disturbance in the developmental period where in cellular and structural formation are.
   Or it may be a degenerative process such as the lipordosis, Schüller's disease or Greenfield's disease. Management is only symptomatic.

SYRINGOMYELIA

Syringomyelia is a chronic myelopathy characterized by the presence of long cavities in the central part of spinal cord. It is sometimes idiopathic or developmental, arising due to the abnormal closure of central canal in the spinal cord in the embryo. It is normally associated with other cerebrovertebro developmental abnormalities. Syringomyelia can occur independent of anomalies of the base of the skull when it is called as noncommunicating syringomyelia.

Incidence and Clinical Presentation

It occurs more in males than in females. Clinical presentation starts in the 3rd or 4th decade of life. They may be progressing in nature like

- Vibration of feet
- Deep tendon reflex is lost
- Subcutaneous edema
- Painless ulcers in the hands
- Hypertrophy of hands and tongue
- Bladder and bowel dysfunction
- Pain in the shoulder and neck
- Osteoporesis without pain.

Diagnosis is done by

- Myelography
- MRI

Management

No specific treatment but symptomatic. But radiation can relieve the pain, when hydrocephalus is present shunting can be useful. Posterior fosssa decompression with removal of posterior rim of foramen magnum and arches of atlas and axis may be useful.

Nursing Management

Nursing management is directed towards the relief of symptoms. If the patient is undergoing surgery, preparation and postoperative care is necessary.

14

Traumatic Conditions of Nervous System

HEAD INJURY

Head injury is a term used to refer an injury to skull, the brain or both structures that is sufficient to get the attention of medical consultation and which interferes the person's normal activities.

Craniocerebral trauma refers to injury to the bony cranial vault or to the brain.

The head injury can be:

- Direct injury
- Indirect injury
- Open head injury
- Closed head injury
- Coup injury
- Countrecoup injury
- Missile injury.

Head Injuries can be Classified as

1. Scalp injuries
   - Contusion
   - Abrasion
   - Laceration.
2. Skull injuries
   - Linear fracture
   - Comminuted fracture
   - Depressed fracture
   - Basal skull fracture
   - Cranial fracture
   - Facial fracture
   - Meningeal tears

- Logorrhea
- Rhinorrhea
- Postnasal drip.

3. Cerebral injuries
   - Concussion
   - Contusion
   - Laceration
   - Brainstem injury.
4. Intracranial hemorrhage
   - Epidural hematoma
   - Subarachnoid hematoma
   - Subdural hematoma
   - Intracerebral hematoma.

Pathophysiology

It is very vast and varies in each case. Minor injuries to scalp alone has least pathology. Severe injuries to scalp can injure the brain, then infection, and also may bleed which can have all signs of increased intracranial pressure and infection.

The head injury can be:

a. Primary head injury
b. Secondary head injury

The *primary head injury* is the direct result of the dynamic mechanism that caused the direct tissue disturbances. The injury can be focal or diffuse. But the effect of injury on his cerebral tissue is a direct result of initial insult. It can cause concussion, contusion or laceration. There may be ischemia, infarction and necrotic areas. Loss of autoregulatory control, increased cerebral blood flow, and changes in the efficiency of blood-brain barrier causes brain edema which can show the signs and symptoms of increased intracranial pressure. If these initial problems are not treated in time, they will lead to secondary head injury.

Secondary head injury: The complications arose from the inefficiently treated primary head injury may be named as secondary head injury. The complication may be systemic hypotension, hypoxemia, increased intracranial pressure, cerebral edema, respiratory problems, infections and so on which may lead to death, if, not handled in time.

SPECIFIC HEAD INJURIES AND ITS MANAGEMENT

Scalp Injuries

The scalp injuries may be:
- Abrasion
- Contusion
- Laceration.

Diagnosis is done by

Physical inspection and skull X-ray.

Treatment

- Abrasion—No specific treatment
- Contusion—Cold applications
- Laceration—Explore sterile glowed hand to see any foreign body and sutures if needed.

Injury or Fracture of Skull

The classification of skull injury may be:
- Linear fracture
- Comminuted fracture
- Depressed fracture
- Compound fracture.

Basal skull fracture—This is more serious as 75 percent of basal skull fractures involve the petrous portion of temporal bone and frontal and temporal bones of the skull.

Diagnosis

1. X-ray of the skull
2. Physical findings—They can be:

   In anterior fossa fracture
   - Rhinorrhea, CSF with blood
   - Subconjunctival hemorrhage
   - Periorbital ecchymosis.

   In middle fossa
   - Otorrhea
   - Hemosympanum
   - Conductive hearing loss
   - Facial nerve palsy
   - Battle's signs (Ecchymous over mastoid bone usually seen after 24 to 36 hours of the injury).

Treatment

Depends upon the type and severity of the fracture
1. Simple linear fracture—No specific treatment.
2. Depressed fracture—Surgical intervention to elevate the depressed bone, and debride the underlying structures of bone fragment.
3. Depressed compound or comminuted fracture—Craniotomy and removal of fractured bone fragments with cranioplasty immediately or in 2nd stage of treatment.
4. Basal skull fracture—Antibiotics and maximum rest is advised.
5. CSF leakage—Automatic resolution is expected in 7 to 10 days. If continues, craniotomy and repair of dural tear is done.

Summary of Skull Fractures

They are:
1. Tears of dura with or without CSF leakage.
2. Contusion or laceration injuries to underlying brain from displacement of bone parts.
3. Contusion or laceration of cranial nerves.
4. Infection of the different parts of brain and meninges.

Nursing Management

The objectives of nursing management are:
- Frequent assessment of neurological signs
- Early recognition of complications
- Control of cerebral edema and increased ICP.

Patient who requires surgery will be managed with same nursing protocols as for a craniotomy.

Patient with basal skull fractures to be:
- Instructed not to blow the nose
- Never do suction through nasal passage
- Watch for facial palsy, deafness, nasal dribling, ecchymosis of temporal bone.

Cerebral Injuries

Concussion

It is a clinical diagnosis that describes transient, temporary, neurogenic dysfunction caused by brain trauma. It can be mild or severe.

Mild Concussion Symptoms

- Temporary neurological dysfunction without loss of consciousness
- Temporary dazing
- Retrograde amnesia.

Severe Concussion Symptoms

- Temporary neurological deficits with a period of unconsciousness
- Retrograde amnesia, traumatic amnesia (retrograde-traumatic amnesia).

Postconcussional Symptoms

These are the symptoms which occur as a sequelae of concussion. They include

- Headache
- Dizziness
- Nervousness
- Irritability
- Insomnia
- Poor concentration
- Difficulty in abstract thinking
- Difficulty in judgement
- Avoidance of crowd
- Loss of inhibitions.

Nursing Management

- Prevention of complication
- Advicing them to report the symptoms early.

Intracranial Hemorrhage (Fig. 14.1)

It can be:

1. Extradural—Under the periosteum and dura mater
2. Subdural—It is between the dura mater and arachnoid layer
3. Subarachnoid—Under the arachnoid mater
4. Intracerebral—It is the bleeding into the cerebral substance.

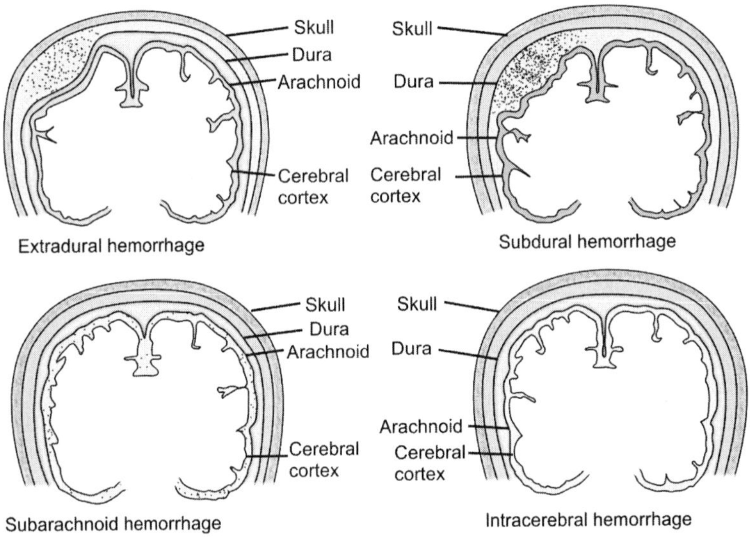

Fig. 14.1: Types of intracranial hemorrhage

Extradural Hematoma

It is also known as an epidural hematoma which refers to a bleeding into potential space between the inner side of skull and the dura mater. It is usually accompanied by skull fracture.

The most common site for fracture is thin, squamous position of the temporal bone, under which is located the middle meningeal artery and vein. A lacerated middle meningeal artery is the cause of bleeding and hematoma. There can be a laceration of superior sagittal sinus which bleeds into the space.

Signs and Symptoms

- Loss of memory, unconsciousness
- Drowsiness
- Confusion to coma
- Headache
- Vomiting
- Dilated-fixed pupils
- Deep respiration-shallow
- Bounding pulse

- Decrease in pulse rate
- Increased temperature.

Diagnosis

CT and skull X-ray.

Management

Always surgical intervention is advised.

Subdural Hematoma

Refers to a bleeding between the dura mater and arachnoid layer. As the arachnoid and pia mater adheres closely to the brain, bleeding to subdural space gives immediate and direct pressure on the brain. The bleeding may occur due to

- Rupture of small veins that bridge the subdural space
- Rupture the cerebral arteries (small branches)
- Bleeding from contused and lacerated areas of brain.

Signs and Symptoms

In acute stage: Headache, drowsiness, irritation and confusion Dilated-fixed pupil

In subacute stage: The sign seen in acute stage will be less severe in subacute stage.

In chronic stage: It can develop gradually from minor head injuries. The time between the injury and the symptoms may be months. So the initial injury may not be remembered. The hematoma slowly increases and behaves like a space occupying lesion.

Signs and Symptoms

- Headache—increase in severity
- Confusion
- Drowsiness
- Seizure
- Hemiparesis.

The other cause for subdural hematoma is normal aging. The atrophy of cerebrum causes separation of cortex from the dura. So the fragile bridging veins are more prone to tear and rupture when a light blow to the skull or a fall on the floor. The same can happen in chronic alcoholic patients.

Diagnosis

- CT scan
- Angiogram if CT not available.

Treatment/Management

In minor case medical treatment is recommended. If the hematoma is large enough, the surgical evacuation is done. Surgical procedure done are either a burrhole and evacuation of hematoma or craniotomy and evacuation.

SUBARACHNOID HEMORRHAGE

It is defined as bleeding into the space under the arachnoid mater of meninges.

Causes may be

- Primary hypertensive hemorrhage
- Ruptured cerebral aneurysm
- Ruptured arteriovenous malformation
- Head injury.

Signs and Symptoms

- Patient may be asymptomatic, alert with minimal headache
- Slight nuchal rigidity, with no neurological deficits
- Drowsy or confused
- May have mild focal deficits
- Stupor
- Mild to severe hemiparesis
- Deep coma, decerebrating.

Management

Management can be medical, surgical according to the causes. Nursing management can be discussed as follows:

- Patient is put on complete bedrest
- Kept in single room with natural and artificial lights

- Indirect light is used while nursing the patient
- Head end of the bed is elevated 30 to 45 degrees
- Patient is to be turned every two hours
- Back care is given gently
- Neurological signs to be recorded hourly
- Vital signs to be recorded frequently
- Patient should be cautioned against coughing and sneezing
- External stimuli to be minimized
- Visitors are limited to immediate family members, that also two at a time
- No enema given
- But constipation is avoided
- Analgesics are given to prevent or treat headaches
- Observe for any seizure activity
- Specific nursing care to be given according to the cause of SAH.

SPINAL CORD INJURY

The spinal cord injury is usually associated with vertebral column injury. It may be appreciated to remember the anatomy of the vertebral column and spinal cord here. The vertebral canal of 33 vertebrate becomes continuously to make a canal like structure which accommodates the spinal cord. The bony part of the vertebrate acts as a protective structure to the spinal cord as the skull does for the brain.

Causes

The injury to the vertebrate may be due to a road accident, fall from height or during a sport activity. The injury can cause a fracture to the vertebrae. The fracture can be

- Simple fracture
- Compression fracture
- Comminuted fracture.

The mechanisms of vertebral fracture are:

- Acceleration and deceleration
- Deformation
- Axial loading
- Penetrating wounds.

Forces involved may be:

- Flexion
- Extension
- Rotation.

These different type of injuries to vertebral column can injure the spinal cord.

Management

The management starts from the place of incident and from the time of the incident.

Immediate Care

While transferring the patient, use firm structure of any improvised method to prevent the further injury to vertebral column and spinal cord.

If the patient has difficulty in breathing, give oxygen or mouth to mouth respiration if oxygen is not available. Prevent or treat any open wound and bleeding to prevent shock and hypovolemia.

While transferring take all precautions not to change the vehicle frequently but keep the patient on a firm board and board should be shifted if needed, not the patient.

In the hospital

- Draw the blood for all investigation and send to the lab on emergency basis
- Monitor the vital signs
- Keep the IV line patent
- Hypovolemia is corrected with IV fluids after receiving the investigation report
- Further diagnosis is done by doing X-ray.

Signs and symptoms may vary according to the area of injury. Common clinical features are:

1. *Spinal shock:* It is a state of transient reflex loss below the level of lesion known as spinal shock. This syndrome may start immediately after the injury and may last for weeks even for months.

   It may result in

   - Loss of motor tone and decreased venous return resulting in hypotension

- Bradycardia because of loss of sympathetic control
- Bladder and bowel dysfunction, initially retention of urine and feces, later may go for incontinence
- Loss of temperature control.

2. *Sensory loss:* There may be loss of sensation of pain, temperature, pressure and touch below the level of injury.
3. *Paralysis:* Quadriplegia or paraplegia can occur according to area of injury.
4. *Bradycardia:* Where there is injury to cervical area, the phrenic nerve is affected and can have changes in respiratory pattern.

Nursing Management of Patients with Spinal Cord Injury

Nursing management can be discussed as follows:

1. *Respiratory system*

   Assess for airway, breathing and circulation quickly. If needed administer O_2 by mask or introducing endotrachial tube. While passing endotrachial tube do not flex or hyperextend the neck as it can damage the cord further. Later do suctioning if needed. But do not do suctioning forcefully. Chest exercises are done frequently to clear the secretions. The accumulation of secretion can cause pneumonia which can cause death.
2. *Circulatory system*
   - Assess for any other injury to any major organs or vessels. As the patient may have the spinal injuries of different region, he may not be able to feel pain so close observation for hypotension rapid pulse or cold clammy skin to be watched as they indicate the internal bleeding. If any of the above said signs are present to be treated immediately with IV fluids even with blood transfusion.
   - Low potassium level can cause cardiac arrhythmias. So electrolytes are assessed frequently and corrected accordingly.
   - Thrombophlebitis and deep vein thrombosis to be assessed frequently to prevent them active and passive movements are given to the extremities.
   - Thigh high elastic stockings can be applied to improve the return flow of blood to the heart.
   - Watch for orthostatic hypotension. Sudden raising of patient's head or even head end of the bed to be avoided to prevent orthostatic hypotension.

3. *Pain*
   Initially the patient may feel pain at the level of injury and no pain is felt below the level of injury. As the spinal shock resolves, some sensations become apparent if the lesion is incomplete. Pain can be managed by analgesics, nerve blocks, biofeedback. But none of them are completely successful in the long-term treatment.
4. *Skin care*
   - Decubitic ulcers are common problem as the patient is immobilized. It is prevented by change in the position in a possible way:
   - Back care is given frequently
   - Bony prominents should be given special attention
   - Patient with overweight or underweight to be given special care to prevent pressure sore
   - Special beds can be provided if possible/needed.
5. *Genitourinary system*
   Urinary retention followed by urinary incontinence, infection and stone formation are the anticipated problems of urinary tract. Care can be given by intake and output chart record and maintain the fluid intake. Bladder assessment is done to determine the line of management. Bladder management should be with the objectives of prevention of further damage to the urinary tract and to provide the patient maximum continent.
6. *Gastrointestinal system*
   The neural innervation, located in the lower intestinal wall is usually not greatly affected by spinal cord injury. Still disabilities can occur like inability to control the anal sphincter, decreased sensation of fullness in the lower bowel. In order to have normal defecation, help the patient to have normal diet with needed roughage and fluid. This planning should be individually tailored as the physiology of GI tract in each individual is different, specially after cord injury.
7. *Sexuality*
   Sexual function is controlled by spinal levels S2, S3 and S4. So lesions involved in this area can cause problems in ejaculation or orgasm. In woman regardless the type of lesion, lacks sensation

during sexual intercourse. They can become pregnant and have vaginal delivery if the pelvic measurements are adequate. Early cesarean section is advised to prevent any complication of delayed labor.

8. *Nutrition*

   It is important to provide nutrition to these patients. Malnutrition can cause unhealthy skin causing bedsores, cardiac arrhythmias, osteoporosis and so on. If patient is unable to take orally, tube feeding or IV fluids are administered.

Special Nursing Care

- Special nursing care to be given if patient is having quadriplegia or paraplegia. Injury to C1 to C8 to L4 can cause paraplegia. One has to assess each nerve for the patient's potentials and design the preventive measures to avoid bedsores and contractures and also to help for early ambulation and rehabilitation.
- If the patient is on cervical skeletal traction, the nurse has the following responsibility:
- Check the frame to see the nuts and bolt are secure.
- Make sure the weights are hanging properly.
- Skin care should be given to prevent bedsores.
- While turning the patient one nurse stands behind the head of the bed and places hands firmly on head and neck, being careful not to flex the head and neck. Second nurse is responsible to move the patient's shoulder. The third nurse is responsible to move patient's hip and legs.
- Be sure to explain the procedure to patient before you start.
- When three nurses are ready, turn the patient in desired position, the nurse who holds the head should keep her hands in place until the patient is supported properly with pillows. If the fraction slips she should provide manual traction until help arrives.

Long-term Treatment

It is important to prepare patient and family to live with the deficits if any. Patient and family should be given the knowledge about the injury, prognosis and possible complications if the care is neglected. Do's and Don'ts should be explained to them according to site of injury, potentials and deficits.

PROLAPSE OF INTERVERTEBRAL DISK (PIVD) (FIG. 14.2)

Prolapse of intervertebral disk is otherwise known as herniated intervertebral disks. Intervertebral disks are fibrocartilagenous substances located between the vertebral bodies from the second cervical vertebra to the sacrum. They vary in size, thickness and shape at different levels of the spine. These disks act as cushion for the vertebrae, help in the movements like, flexion, extension, etc.

So the herniation of the intervertebral disks is the major cause of severe and chronic back pain particularly in the low back region.

Causes for Intervertebral Disk Prolapse

1. Trauma
   - Direct injuries
   - Lifting of heavy objects, slipping
   - Fall on buttocks or back
   - Suppressing sneeze.
2. Degenerative diseases of vertebrae
   - Osteoarthritis
   - Spondylitis.
3. Congenital abnormalities
   - Scoliosis.

Pathology

Degenerative changes or changes due to trauma can occur in the posterior ligaments of the vertebrae. Along with aging, degenerative changes or tears due to injury occur in intervertebral disk also. Then the disk is prone to slip either laterally or centrally into spinal canal, where it encroaches upon nerve roots. This herniation may be spontaneously reduced or reabsorbed but more often it persists as a source of chronic root irritation. The presence of pain depends upon the quantity of disk material herniated into spinal canal, the degree of narrowing of spinal canal, the number of disks involved and the degree of encroachment on nerve roots.

Signs and Symptoms

Lumbar area

1. *Pain:* Low pain radiating to buttock, thigh, one leg, for varying periods. (This is sometimes called sciatica).

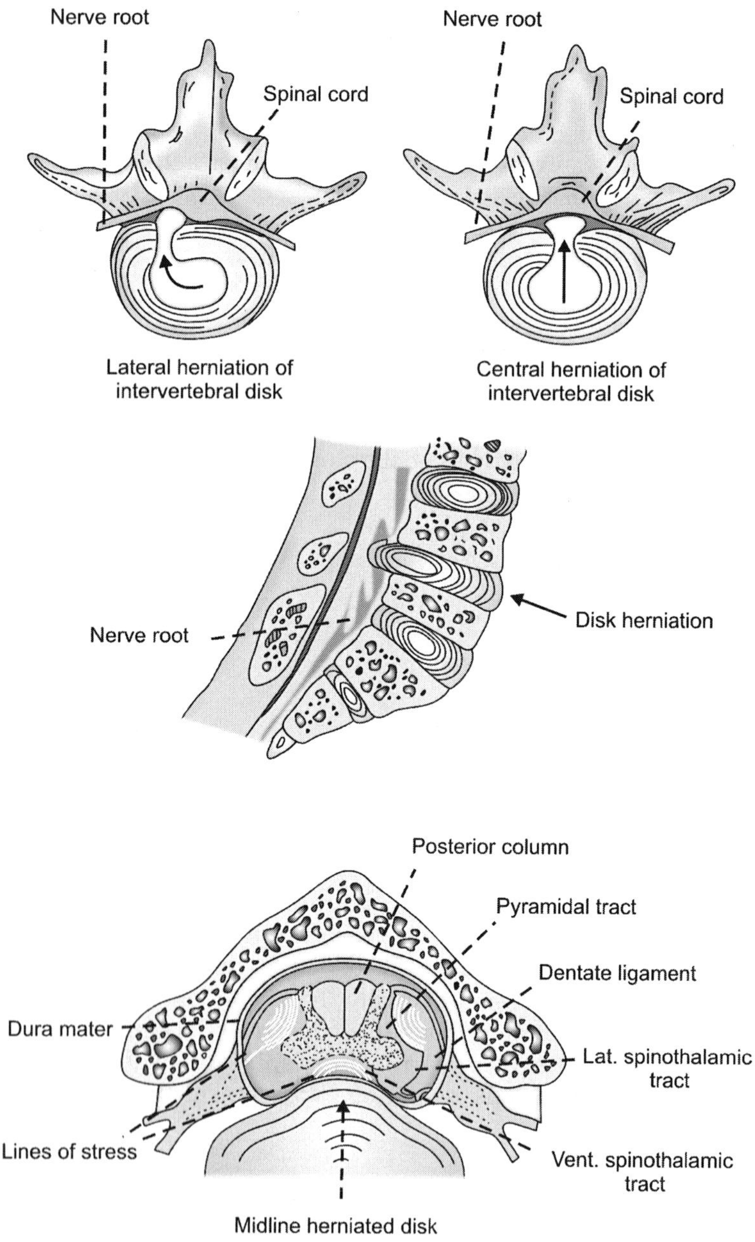

Fig. 14.2: Intervertebral disk prolapse

- Pain from herniated disk is aggravated by coughing, sneezing, straining, stooping, blowing the nose and jarring movement while walking or riding. Pain can be while sitting, or lying or both sitting and lying.

2. *Motor changes*
   - Hypotonia is most common with motor root compression
   - Slight motor weakness
   - Weakness of plantar flexion and dorsiflexion
   - Atrophy of affected muscles can develop
   - Footdrop can be noticed
   - Difficulty in micturation and sexual activity
3. *Sensory changes*
   - Paresthesia in leg and foot
   - Numbness in leg and foot
   - Tenderness of affected disk.
4. *Alterations of reflexes*
   - Knee and ankle reflexes may be absent or diminished depending upon the level of disk herniation.
   - Pain and other symptoms with disk prolapse are recurrent. Remission of acute episodes are probably due to the recession of protruding disk, decreased local edema, relief of root compression and reabsorption of disk exudates.

Cervical Area

1. In lateral herniation pain is in the shoulders, neck and arm. Stiff neck, motor weakness, tenderness locally, weakness of hand, forearm, atrophy of muscle.
2. Paracentral herniation: Pain is mild, insidious, intermittent, weakness of lower extremities, spasticity, difficulty in voiding, sexual activities, reflexes in lower extremities can become hyperactive, and can cause syringomyelia.

Diagnosis is made by

- History
- X-ray, myelogram
- Physical examination.

Management

1. Conservative
2. Surgical.

Conservative Management

- Decrease general activity
- Avoid flexion of spine
- Avoid lifting, bending, twisting
- Use support like brace, collar, etc.
- Use firm mattress while resting or sleeping
- Physiotherapy can be advised
- Skin traction is advised
- Drugs to reduce pain, edema can be given.

Surgical Management

The conservative treatment is given for 2 to 6 weeks. If the repeat X-ray/myelogram does not show any improvement along with no remarkable positive improvement in the signs and symptoms, surgery is advised.

Surgical procedures suggested are:

1. Hemilaminectomy—Excersion of part of posterior arch of vertebral lamina.
2. Anterior cervical discectomy and fusion—Anterior approach to remove the part of disk and to perform a fusion of two vertebra.
3. Bone fusion—Immobilization of two vertebrae by inserting a wedge shaped piece of bone usually taken from the iliac crest of patient's own body.

As a whole, the surgical procedure is called 'laminectomy' which can be named as cervical laminectomy, lumbar laminectomy and thoracic laminectomy, according to the region it is performed.

Nursing Management: During Conservative Management

- Maintain firm mattresses to support the diseased vertebrae.
- Maintain bedrest to avoid any strain on the affected part which can aggravate the symptoms.
- Assess the vital signs frequently.
- Do the neurological assessment frequently.
- Maintain body alignment which decreases stress of irritated muscles.
    i. Small pillow in nape of the neck for cervical disk
    ii. A small pillow under knees and under the head
- Caution the patient against twisting, stretching, straining, etc.

- Encourage the patient to do motion exercise in the bed.
- Encourage breathing exercises.
- Provide enough roughage to prevent constipation.
- Provide all personal hygiene like, body bath, mouth care, hair care, etc.
- Give back care with special care to all dependent areas of the body.
- If patient is with cervical collar, see that collar is in position to support the affected area.
- If skin traction is applied ensure the traction is in position to give enough traction to keep the body in alignment.
- Patient should not be allowed to strain during defecation, constipation to be avoided.
- If sensation is lost care to be taken to prevent burns.

Nursing management for patient with surgical treatment

- Preoperative management as usual.
- Routine preoperative care like shaving, patient teaching, is done.
- Specially the patient to be explained about the procedure.
- Expected outcome should be explained as the surgery does not always relieve the pain permanently.
- Explanation should be given about the importance of complete rest for few hours and restricted movement for few days or months.

Postoperative management

- Patient should be received with firm mattress.
- Keep the bed flat.
- If cervical laminectomy is done a small pillow can be given under the nape of neck.
- For lumbar laminectomy small pillow can be placed under the head and one may be placed under the knees periodically.
- Reposition of patient can be done with proper precaution to keep the body in good alignment.
- Assess the vital signs frequently.
- Neurological assessment is done frequently. Especially movements in extremities and feeling of touch in legs.
- For cervical laminectomy patient's arms and shoulders are taken care frequently for any deficits.
- Do not allow the patient to turn or strain himself.
- Can be encouraged to move the extremities in the bed.

- Deep breathing can be encouraged.
- Intake and output chart is maintained and nutrition is maintained.
- Observe the wound for any leakage or wetting.
- Drugs can be given to relieve pain, inflammation or infection.
- For cervical laminectomy patient, sore throat is expected so that vescoris lignocaine can be given.
- Lumbar laminectomy patient is allowed out of bed on 2nd and 3rd day.
- Sit for minimum time for at least one week.
- On discharge on 6th or 7th day patient can be allowed to sit in hard, and straight chair.
- Cervical laminectomy patient is evaluated for dizziness before getting out of bed.
- Cervical laminectomy—the cervical collar is used till the alignment is complete.
- Patient is asked not to pull or push with hand for at least few weeks.

Special considerations in spinal fusion

- The immobilization is advised for a long period to allow healing the fusion.
- To allow the immobilization body cast may be used in thoracic and lumbar fusion and cervical collar in cervical fusion.
- In anterior cervical diskectomy and fusion, injuries to soft tissues like oesophages or larynx can occur. If so laryngeal edema can occur causing difficulty in coughing, breathing. So endotracheal tube is inserted to make the respiration easy.

On discharge

- Instruct not to go for any vigorous activity like
  - Bending
  - Stretching
  - Lifting heavy objects should be avoided for few weeks and to be started gradually
- Use firm bed while sleeping
- Use only small pillows
- Do not ride the vehicles
- Do not travel on bad roads
- Any slight pain should be taken care by taking rest.

15

Vascular Diseases

ANEURYSM

Definition

A cerebral aneurysm is a round sacular dilatation of the arterial wall that develops as a result of weakness of the wall. These aneurysms can be of different types (Figs 15.1A to C):

1. Berry aneurysms—Which has stem and a neck
2. Giant aneurysm—Which has no neck
3. Mycotic, septic emboli from infection may lead to aneurysms
4. Charcot-Bouchard aneurysms
5. Traumatic aneurysm.

The usual size of the aneurysm is 1 cm but it can go up to 5 cm rarely.

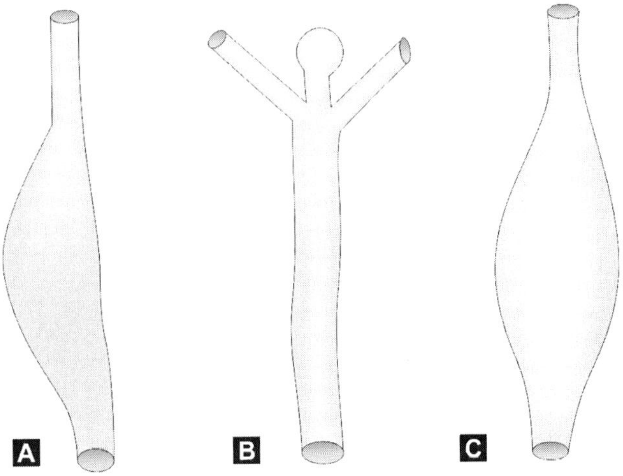

Figs 15.1A to C: Types of aneurysm (A) Sacular, (B) Berry, and (C) Fusiform

Possible Causes are

1. Hypertension
2. Polycystic disease
3. Congenital defects in the cerebral arteries
4. Trauma after head injury.

Pathology

Rupture causes bleeding to subarachnoid, subdural or intracranial areas. Signs and symptoms of stroke is increased ICP will be the general pathology. The specific symptoms will be associated with location of hemorrhage and the degree of increased intracranial pressure.

Signs and Symptoms

Before Rupture

- Headache
- Lethargy
- Neck pain
- Dysfunction of optic and oculomotor nerve.

After Rupture

- Severe headache
- Visual disturbances
- Irritation
- Stiff neck
- Posture—Kernig's and Brudzinski's signs.

Diagnosis

- History and physical examination
- Lumbar puncture
- CT scan
- Cerebral angiogram.

Management

Medical management till the patient is fit for surgery. If the patient is fit for surgery, craniotomy and clipping of aneurysm can be done.

Nursing Management

Before Surgery

- Patient should be put on complete bedrest
- Vital signs to be recorded frequently and give the care to keep the vital signs stable by appropriate IV fluids and position
- Monitor the neurological signs to look for the signs of increased intracranial pressure.
- All the general nursing care to be given like prevention of
  - Infection especially, systemic
  - Bedsore
  - Bladder and bowel irregularities
  - Nutritional deficiency
  - Contractures.

After Surgery

- Keep the patient in quite environment
- Watch for any signs of increased ICP
- Close observation for any neurological deficits
- Avoid constipation
- Strict intake and output chart
- Observation for any seizure
- Vital signs to be checked and recorded to see any rebleeding occurs.

General Nursing Care Includes

- Personal hygiene
- Prevent bedsore
- Prevent systemic infection
- Prevent local infection
- Prevent respiratory complication/infection
- Prevent nutritional deficiency
- Prevent urinary tract infections and incontinence
- Prevent constipation.

ARTERIOVENOUS MALFORMATION (AVM)

An arteriovenous malformation is condition in which a tangled array of dilated vessels form an abnormal communication network between the arterial and venous system. In this condition, the arterial blood is directly shunted into a vein without going to capillaries. This may be small or big, deep or superficial. The deep-seated AVM may be in ventricles and affect the choroids plexus and causes hydrocephalus.

Pathology

1. Ischemia in affected areas which can cause seizure, stroke
2. Gliosis can occur because of prolonged ischemia
3. Compression of local tissue and deficits accordingly
4. Hemorrhage: Bleeding can be of small quantity without any neurological deficits. Major bleeding can occur causing increased intracranial pressure and its complications.
5. Noncommunicating hydrocephalus: The downward pressure from the tortuous vein can obstruct the ventricular system, then preventing normal flow of cerebrospinal fluid.

Signs and Symptoms

1. Hemorrhage and associated symptoms
2. Seizure activity
3. Headache
4. Transient attacks of syncope
5. Dizziness
6. Visual disturbances
7. Intellectual impairment if the AVM is in frontal lobe.

Diagnosis is done by

- Angiography
- CT scan
- Skull films
- Electroencephalography
- Lumbar puncture.

Management

Medical, if surgery is not advisable.

Embolization

It is done when the lesion is inaccessible. This technique as perceived by Luessenhop in early 1960s. The procedure involves introducing small silastic beads into internal carotid artery by means of a catheter which enters the malformation. This procedure helps to distract the lesions.

Surgical Management

If the AVM is accessible a craniotomy and complete excision of the lesion is advisable. Preoperative and postoperative care is as of any craniotomy unless any special condition are associated with AVM.

Nursing Management

Nursing management is also of any cranial surgery, i.e.
- Observe for any signs of increased intracranial pressure
- Observe for any seizure activity
- Observe for any neurological deficit
- Do all the general nursing care like prevention of
  - bedsore
  - nutritional deficit
  - systemic or local interaction
  - bladder and bowel problems
  - contractures and
  - footdrop if the patient is bedridden.

16

Tumors of Nervous System

TUMOR

Tumor is called as neoplasm, a new growth of tissue characterized by progressive uncontrolled proliferation of cells. The tumor may be localized or invasive, benign or malignant. A tumor may be named for its location, for its cellular makeup or for the person who first identified it.

BRAIN TUMOR

Brain tumor is a neoplasm of the intracranial portion of the central nervous system that is usually invasive but does not spread beyond the cerebrospinal axis.

When one looks at the percentage of brain tumors of all cancer deaths, it is very small. But in terms of human suffering and disability caused by brain tumors, it is a major concern for nurses, caring for these patients.

Classification of Brain Tumors

They are classified in different ways by different people.
They are as follows:

1. Malignant and benign
2. Intradural and extradural
3. Histological according to cells from which the tumors arise.

Malignant and Benign

As the names indicate, the malignant has poor prognosis and benign is considered as curable. But the benign tumors which are surgically inaccessible or located on a vital organ will be left alone for longer time can grow indefinitely. This growth can cause raised intracranial pressure, neurological deficits, herniation syndromes and finally death. And also there is a possibility that tumors can convert to more histologically malignant types as they develop.

Intra-axial and Extra-axial Brain Tumors

Tumors originating from brain substance are termed intra-axial tumors and affect the brain by invasions and infiltration. Extra-axial tumors originate in the skull, meninges, cranial nerves and pituitary and the congenital cells at rest. Compression of the brain is the mode by which extra-axial tumors affect the brain.

Histological Classification of Brain Tumor

A. Intrinsic tumors—They are again divided into
   1. Gliomas
      a. Astrocytoma—Grade I and II are low grade
Grade III is malignant
Grade IV is glioblastoma (high grade malignant tumor)
      b. Oligodendrogliomas
      c. Ependymoma
      d. Mixed gliomas
   2. Medulloblastoma

B. Tumors arising from supporting structures
   a. Meningioma
   b. Neuroma
   c. Schwannoma

C. Developmental (congenital tumors)
   a. Craniopharyngeomas
   b. Dermoids

D. Pituitary tumors
   a. Chromophobic or functioning and nonfunctioning
   b. Eosinophilic
   c. Basophilic

E. Metastatic tumors
   a. Lung, breast
   b. Malignant melanomas.

Definitions of Tumors of Different Histological Origin

Gliomas: It is a type of tumor originating from neuroglial cells. It can be of brain or spinal cord.

Astrocytoma: It is a type of gliomas from astrocytes.

Glioblastoma: It is a type of gliomas otherwise called astrocytoma Grade III and IV arising from cerebral hemispheres.

Oligodendrogliomas: It is a type of glioma arising from oligodendroglia.

Ependymoma: It is a tumor arising from the lining of ventricles of brain (Ependymol cells). It can give signs of hydrocephalus.

Medulloblastoma: Rapid growing tumors of neuroepithelial origin occurring in childhood and usually seen near 4th ventricles of the brain from cerebellum.

Neuromas: It is a benign tumor composed of fibrous tissue and nerve fibers. It may be soft or hard. Pain radiating from the tumor may be intermittent or continuous. Pain can reach the periphery.

Meningioma: They are tumors of the membranes (meninges) covering the brain and spinal cord. They grow often slowly, but are highly vascular. Commonly seen on the convexity of dura mater of the brain. It can cause bone erosion and compression of brain tissue. It can occur after head injury.

Schwannoma: They are tumors of Schwann cells around the nerves, commonly seen from 8th cranial nerve.

Hemangioblastoma: Tumor arises from the brain or spinal cord consisting of proliferate cells around blood vessels. They are vascular.

Craniopharyngioma: It is congenital sellar/suprasellar tumor, appearing most often in children and adolescents, that arise in cells derived from Rathke's pouch or the hypophyseal stalk. The lesion, a solid or cystic body ranging in size from 1 to 8 cm, may expand into the third ventricle or temporal lobe, frequently becomes calcified. This tumor may interfere with pituitary function damage optic chiasm, disrupt hypothalamic control of autonomic nervous system and result in hydrocephalus. Development tumor after puberty can cause amenorrhea in women, loss of potency in men.

Other names are ameloblastoma, pituitary adamantinoma, Rathke's pouch tumor.

Pituitary Tumor

Chromophobic: It is a nonsecreting tumor of pituitary gland.

Basophilic: It is a secreting tumor producing adrenocorticotropic hormones causing hyperplasia of adrenal gland. This tumor can grow fast causing enlargement of sella.

Eosinophilic: Secreting tumor causing extraproduction of gland's hormone.

Difference in Brain Tumor in Children and Adults

In children from newborn to 16 years the incidence of brain tumors differ with about two-third of all childhood brain tumors are located in posterior fossa (Table 16.1).

Table 16.1: Different brain tumors in children

Types	*Percentage of total primary childhood tumors*
Medulloblastomas	30
Astrocytomas	30
Ependymoma	12
Craniopharyngioma	10
Optic pathway gliomas	05
Miscellaneous	13

Pathophysiology of Brain Tumors

A brain tumor will usually grow until it encounters a more rigid structure, such as bone or falx cerebri. The size of the tumor enlarges because of cell proliferation or as a result of necrosis, fluid accumulation, hemorrhage, or accumulation of by-products of degeneration within the mass.

Tumor affect the brain through compression, invasion and infiltration. These mechanisms precipitate pathophysiological changes in the brain resulting in some or all of the following findings:

1. Cerebral edema
2. Increased intracranial pressure
3. Focal neurological deficits
4. Seizures
5. Alteration in normal pituitary function
6. Obstruction of flow of cerebrospinal fluid.

These pathophysiological changes cause serious problems in individuals which can lead to temporary neurological deficits, permanent neurological deficits or even death.

1. *Cerebral edema*: Cerebral edema creates signs and symptoms of increased intracranial pressure that include
   - Deterioration of level of consciousness
   - Loss of decreased reactions of the pupils to the direct light reflex
   - Unequal papillary size
   - Loss or decreased functional eye movement
   - Loss or deterioration of motor function
   - Loss or deterioration of sensory function
   - Changes in respiratory function
   - Changes in vital signs with decreased pulse rate, increased BP and widening of pulse pressure.
2. *Increased cranial pressure:* In an adult most brain tumors are located in supratentorial region. Without definite treatment of these neoplasms, intracranial displacement will continue until brainstem-cerebellar herniation occurs through the foramen magnum. The vital centers of the brainstem then become compressed and death occurs.
3. *Focal neurological deficits:* Cerebral tissue is highly specialized. Any disturbance by compression, invasion or edema will result in functional deficits. Cranial nerves III, IV and VI are frequently affected by expanding supratentorial tumors, compression of blood vessels produces a diminished blood supply and possible ischemia to the areas supplied by the particular vessels. Stretching or traction on a vessel can cause rupture and subsequent hemorrhage. This hemorrhage cause further intracranial pressure symptoms.
4. *Seizure activity:* Cerebral edema and alterations in the normal electric potential of the cell caused by the tumor results in hyperactive cells. This hyperactivity produces abnormal paroxysmal discharge or seizure activity that may be grand mal or focal.
5. *Changes in the pituitary function:* These tumors are usually from anterior lobe of pituitary gland. Adenomas of pituitary gland directly affect the pituitary function. The craniopharyngiomas, some meningiomas and aneurysms located near the pituitary-hypothalamus can also produce endocrine imbalance.

The following is a list of major secretions and their functions which can be affected by the different above said tumors.

- Thyroid stimulating hormone- releasing factor (TRF) causes release of thyroid stimulating hormone (TSH).
- Corticotropin-releasing factor (CRF) causes release of adrenocorticotropin.
- Growth hormone-releasing hormone factor (GHF) causes release of growth hormone.
- Leutinizing hormone-release factor (LRF) causes release of leutinizing hormone.
- Follicle stimulating hormone-release factor (FRF) causes release of follicle stimulating hormone.
- Prolactin inhibitory factor (PIF) causes inhibition of prolactin secretion.

So, any alteration in any of these pituitary secretions result in major disruption of body function causing conditions like gigantism, acromegaly, Cushing's syndrome or hypopituitarism.

6. *Obstructions of flow of cerebrospinal fluid:* The cerebrospinal fluid is secreted in the lateral ventricles of the brain. From there it escapes to 3rd and to 4th ventricles and then to the subarachnoid spaces of spinal cord and around the brain. Finally, it is absorbed in the subarachnoid villi of meninges. So any tumor obstructing the pathway of CSF can cause obstruction of the free flow. This causes accumulation of CSF above the tumor/obstruction which causes hydrocephalus and subsequent symptoms of increased intracranial pressure.

Signs and Symptoms of Brain Tumors

General symptoms

- Headache
- Vomiting
- Papilledema
- Personality changes.

Signs and Symptoms Related to Tumor Area

Frontal lobe tumors

- Inappropriate behavior
- Inattentiveness
- Inability to concentrate
- Emotional liability

- Impairment of recent memory
- Difficulty with abstraction
- Flat effect.

Parietal Lobe Tumors
- Decreased tactile sensitivity
- Loss of right left discrimination
- Construction apraxia
- Seizure activity.

Temporal Lobe Tumors
- Hallucination—auditory, visual, olfactory
- Receptive aphasia
- Irritability
- Depression
- Poor judgment
- Childish behavior.

Occipital Lobe Tumors
- Visual disturbance
- Visual hallucination.

Cerebellum Tumors
- Ataxia, incoordination.

Brainstem Tumors
- Dysphagia
- Vomiting
- Motor/sensory tract deficits.

Pituitary Tumors
- Gigantism
- Acromegaly
- Cushing's syndrome
- Hypopituitarism
- Changes in metabolisms of fat, carbohydrate and water.

Midbrain Tumors
- Cerebellar symptoms
- Deafness
- Decreased light reflex.

Ventricular Tumors
- Headache
- Vomiting
- Signs of increased intracranial pressure.

Investigations

1. History and physical examination
2. Visual field and fundoscopic examination
3. Skull films
4. Computed tomography
5. Electroencephalogram
6. Cerebral angiography
7. Lumbar puncture
8. Magnetic resource image
9. Endocrinal studies.

Management of Patient with Tumors of Nervous System

Once it is diagnosed as brain tumor, it can be treated by three methods: surgery, radiation and chemotherapy. The methods can be used alone or in combination. Selection of these modalities depend on the size, type and location of the tumor.

Chemotherapy

Drugs used are:

1. Dexamethasone (Decadron)—To reduce the cerebral edema
2. Phenytoin—To prevent or treat the seizure activity
3. Antiedematic—glycerol, mannitol
4. Antibiotics.

Nursing Care of Patients who are with Chemotherapy

1. Record the vital signs to look for any signs of increased intracranial pressure.
2. Observe any other symptoms of increased intracranial pressure like headache, vomiting.
3. Watch for any seizure activity and keep the record.
4. Use all support strategies to keep the patient fit and fine.

The common surgical procedures done for the patients with tumors of nervous system:

1. Craniotomy of different regions, depending upon the site of tumor
2. Shunt of different types in case of noncommunicating tumors causing hydrocephalis
3. Laser surgeries
4. Use of gamma knife

5. Interventional radiotherapy
6. Burrhole for biopsy.

This nursing care of patient with increased intracranial pressure and seizure activity is discussed in concerned chapters.

Preoperative and postoperative care in general and same specific observations are discussed in this handbook.

PRE- AND POSTOPERATIVE CARE OF PATIENTS UNDERGOING NEUROSURGERIES

Preoperative Management

The surgery can be planned or unplanned. For the planned surgery, the preoperative care starts on the day the patient comes to the hospital for the first time. The preoperative period can be divided into:

- Care given in outpatient department
- Care given from the day of admission till the day of surgery
- On the day of surgery till the patient reaches the operation theater
- In the operation theater till the surgery is started.

1. In the outpatient department the following steps are taken:
   a. History
   b. Investigation
   c. Make the patient fit for surgery; physically, mentally financially and socially
   d. Here the family also is given support.
2. On admission the patient is given physical orientation. Orientation to the routine of the ward, orientation to the staff. Patient is given information about the nature of surgical procedure, possible complications if the patient is in a position to understand.
3. The day of surgery—consent, physical preparation, keeping ready all the investigation report, premedication keeping ready the preoperative check list, and accompanying the patient till the operation theater.
4. In the operation theater, the nurse receives the patient with all records, handover the patient to the anesthetist and his/her team.

Intraoperative Care

Nursing care can be under the following heading:

- Prevention of hypotension
- Prevention of hypothermia and hyperthermia
- Prevention of hyperventilation

- Prevention of air embolism if the patient is in sitting position
- Prevention of any type of burns when diathermy is used.

Postoperative Care

After surgery the patient is taken to the recovery room or to the neurosurgical intensive care unit. Here, the environment allows for close monitoring to meet any emergency. Here, the nurse should have or obtain the necessary documents like:

- Postoperative notes
- History of preoperative neurological status of patient
- Current (postoperative) baseline neurological assessment
- Review the postoperative order.

Nursing care following craniotomy is with the objective of:

- Frequent monitoring and recording of neurological signs to identify the signs of increased intracranial pressure.
- Frequent monitoring of vital signs to prevent the causes for increased intracranial pressure.
- Look for any seizure activity.
- Observe for any neurological deficit.

Care in Postoperative Ward

Continue the observations and prepare the patient for discharge. Planning for early rehabilitation is essential, i.e. according to the condition and need for the individual patient.

Special Nursing Care of Patients Undergoing Surgery for Pituitary Tumors

Preoperative

- Daily weight checking
- 24 hours urine volume for 3 consecutive days
- Intake and output chart for 3 days
- If the approach is oral/nasal swab is sent for culture and sensitivity, urine and blood also sent for osmolality.

Postoperative

- Weight to be checked daily
- Strict intake and output chart—watch for negative balance and inform
- Nasal drops to be put.

If nasal pack is there
- Head end to be elevated
- Bedrest to be advised
- Instruct not to sneeze
- Instruct not to cough
- Oral respiration to be advised.

Serum electrolyte and osmolality to be checked and maintained. Urine osmolality and urine electrolytes to be checked.

Special Nursing Care for Patients Undergoing Surgery for CP Angle Tumor

Preoperative Care—Nothing Special

Postoperative care
- No oral feeds till the gag reflex return
- Give exercises for facial muscles to prevent or treat facial palsy
- If facial palsy is there, tarsorrhaphy is done
- Care of the eye is important.

Though the general nursing care of patients with tumors of nervous system is discussed here, the care may be modified in each case as the patient may have any other general health problem along with these conditions. And the care of patients with tumors of the spinal cord is always in line with the care of patients with spinal cord injuries and surgeries which is discussed in the concerned chapters.

OPERATIVE APPROACHES IN NEUROSURGERY

Cranial Surgery

For Supratentorial Tumors

- *Craniotomy:* Depending on the site it can be frontal, temporal, parietal, pterional or occipital or combination of these. Here removal of the bone flap and replacing the bone flap is performed.

For Infratentorial Tumor

- *Craniectomy:* Here removal of the bone without replacement is done. This is for posterior fossa tumors like acoustic schwannoma.
- Depending on the site it can be suboccipital craniectomy, midline, lateral or retromastoid craniectomy.

In some patients bone flap may not be replaced following craniotomy. This is done to increase the space for the brain. In such patients without bone flap care should be taken during nursing to avoid any injury. Defects in the cranium following trauma or surgery can be filled with acrylic (bone like material), this procedure is called cranioplasty.

For Pituitary Tumors

Transphenoidal route to approach pituitary tumors:

Transphenoidal route done through the nose directly called transnasal, transphenoidal or through the upper lip and nose called sublabial transphenoidal. This approach is to reach the sellar and suprasellar areas through the sphenoid sinus approaching from the nose.

Spinal Lesions

Laminectomy

This can be approached from anterior or posterior.

1. *Cervical disk excision:* Anterior cervical approach is preferred.
2. *Lumbar disk:* Posterior approach by laminectomy or hemilaminectomy or fenestration is done.
   - Laminectomy—removal of lamina completely.
   - Hemilaminectomy—removal of the lamina on one side only.
   - Fenestration—is going between two lamina without removing lamina.

   Laminectomy is also done in cervical spondylosis and lumbar canal stenosis for decompression to increase the space in the spinal canal for the neural element.
3. *Laminotomy:* is replacement of lamina following the posterior approach for spine. If the spinal canal is remodeled by replacing the lamina in a different fashion to increase the space in the spinal canal it is called laminoplasty.
4. *Fusion:* Fusion with bone grafts taken from the iliac crest or ribs can be done following removal of vertebral bodies (corpectomy). Plates and screws are used to fix the bones above and below the corpectomy and the bone grafts. This procedure is done when there is spinal instability following trauma or disk diseases or spondylosis or surgeries.

For tuberculosis of the spine: Anteriolateral decompression is done to let out pus. This can be combined with fusion.

5. *Other approaches to the spine:* In the thoracic region anterior approach to the spine can be through the thorax or abdomen. Accordingly it is called transthoracic extra or intrapleural and transabdominal retroperitoneal approach.

17

Neuromuscular Disorders

MUSCULAR DYSTROPHIES

Muscular dystrophy is a group of genetically transmitted diseases characterized by progressive atrophy of symmetric groups of skeletal muscles without evidence of involvement or degeneration of neural tissue. In all forms of muscular dystrophy there is a insidious loss of strength with increasing disability and deformity. But each type differs in the group of muscles affected, the age of onset, the rate of progress and mode of genetic inheritance.

Types of Muscular Dystrophy

1. Duchenne (pseudohypertrophy)	Commonly found
2. Limb-girdle	
3. Facioscapulohumeral (Landouzy-Dejerine)	
4. Becker's muscular dystrophy	Rarely found
5. Distal muscular dystrophy	
6. Ocular myopathy	
7. Myotonic muscular dystrophy.	

Causes

Basic cause is unknown, but appears to be an inborn error of metabolism. Serum creatinine phosphokinase is increased in affected individuals.

Diagnosis is Made by

1. Blood investigation to look for creatinine phosphokinase level
2. Urine analysis for creatinine
3. Electromyography
4. Genetic pedigree.

Duchenne's Muscular Dystrophy

Is an abnormal congenital condition characterized by progressive symmetric, wasting of the leg muscles and pelvic muscles. The disease affects predominantly males and accounts for 50 percent of all muscular dystrophy diseases. It is chromosome linked recessive disease that appears insidiously between 3 and 5 year of age and spreads from the leg and pelvic muscles to the involuntary muscles. Associated muscle weakness produces a waddling gait and pronounced as lordiosis. Muscles rapidly deteriorate and calf muscles become firm and enlarged with fatty deposits. They later develop contractures, difficulty in climbing stairs, often stumble and fall, display wing scapula. Usually by the age of 12, they confine to wheelchair. They may have tachycardia, pulmonary problems, arrhythmias (cardiac), cardiac murmurs.

Diagnosis is done by

- Blood for CPK level, LDH (lactic dehydrogenase)
- Electromyography
- Muscle biopsy
- Urinalysis.

Treatment

- No successful treatment is available
- Orthopedic appliances are used accordingly
- Physical therapy
- Exercises
- Amniocentesis is recommended during pregnancy to detect the sex.

Nursing Care

- Psychological support
- Recommend and encourage physical activities
- Encourage to have peer interactions and social therapies
- Emotional support to family members.

Limb-girdle Dystrophy

This condition transmitted as an autosomal recessive trait characterized by weakness and degeneration of the muscles begins in the shoulder girdle or in pelvic girdle. The condition is progressive since no effective treatment is available. It can be classified as pelvic femoral muscular dystrophy and scapulohumeral muscular dystrophy.

Other forms of muscular dystrophies are rare. As there is no complete cure for these conditions nursing care is only in the direction of supportive. Prevention can be done by termination of pregnancy, if it is diagnosed by scanning during antenatal period of risk groups.

MYASTHENIA GRAVIS (MG)

The name myasthenia comes from Greek meaning muscle weakness and gravis from Latin meaning severe. Thomas Willis, British physician was the first person to describe the disease in 1672.

Definition

Myasthenia gravis is a chronic progressive disease of muscular weakness caused by chemical transmitter acetylcholine deficiency at the point of myoneural junction. As a result, muscle does not receive the motor impulse properly and does not contract well.

The hallmark of the disease are:

- Increased weakness of certain muscles, particularly those of chewing, swallowing and speaking as well as facial and extraocular muscles.
- Partial improvement with rest.
- Dramatic improvement in muscle strength with anticholinesterase drugs.

Epidemiology

- Prevalence of MG is about 0.5 to 14.5 per million.
- Peak incidence of myasthenia gravis is between 20 to 30 years.
- Women are more affected.
- After the age of 40 years the frequency in men and women is about equal.

Etiology

The cause and deficiency of this acetylcholine is not known. The possible explanations of pathological condition have been offered.

1. It is caused by a deficiency of acetylcholine receptor (presynaptic level).
2. It is caused by a disturbance at the end (postsynaptic).
3. This is caused by the defect of abnormality in the muscle fiber itself.
4. There is increasing evidence that the thymus gland plays an important role in autoimmunological process. It also has been suggested that myasthenia gravis is produced by autoimmune mechanism that destroys or inactivates the sensitive receptor substance in the muscle. The abnormal neuromuscular transmission in myasthenia is attributed to the circulating acetylcholine receptor.

Pathophysiology

The pathophysiology of myasthenia gravis is attributed to a defect at the myoneural junction. As an impulse travels down the peripheral nerve, it relies on the release of acetylcholine to transmit the impulse across the myoneural junction to the innervated muscle in order for a contraction to take place. In myasthenia gravis the amount of acetylcholine in the presynaptic membrane is reduced. It is believed that a defect in the presynaptic membrane causes a reduced amount of acetylcholine. There is evidence also that the postsynaptic membrane lacks sufficient receptor sites to use acetylcholine. Both of these reasons contribute to the fact that muscle is not able to contract fully or normally. With repeated stimulation the muscle becomes exhausted and cannot contract at all.

The prognosis without treatment is grave. Until the advent of anticholinesterase therapy most patients died from respiratory insufficiency and less frequently from aspiration.

Eighty percent of myasthenic patient are said to have thymic hyperplasia, 15 percent have thymic tumors. Some evidence is there to suggest that toxic substance produced by the hyperplastic thymus influence the development of myasthenia gravis.

Signs and Symptoms

1. Muscle weakness is the main feature in this disease. First eye muscles will be affected. Patient will have ptosis unilateral or bilateral. There will be difficulty in closing the eyelids.

2. Difficulty in chewing, talking, using the neck muscle, smiling and swallowing will be present. Patient may have to take periods of rest while eating.
3. Voice becomes weak and fades after conversation, diminishes to whisper.
4. Drooping of the shoulder forward and difficulty keeping the arm above his head when combing or fixing the hair will be there.
5. If the hand muscles are involved, writing, sewing and other fine movements will be impaired.
6. The most life-threatening situation arises when intercostal muscles, diaphragm are affected. Breathlessness and respiratory weakness can lead to death.
7. The muscles are strongest in the morning and become exhausted after the use or towards the end of the day.

Diagnosis is Based on

1. History of weakness of muscle.
2. Tensilon test: This is most reliable test. The test is performed by drawing 10 mg of tensilon (edrophonium chloride) into a syringe and administering 2 mg. If any improvement in muscle strength, the remaining 8 mg of the drug is injected.
   Within 30 to 60 seconds of the first dose, most patients with myasthenia gravis will demonstrate a marked, objective improvement, in muscle tone lasting for 4 to 5 mts. A few myasthenia patients will respond only to the larger dose. The test is also a valid tool for differentiating between myasthenia and cholinergic crisis.
3. Blood test: Routine test to ascertain the patient's general health and exclude anemia
   a. Examination for antibodies (titer of acetylcholine receptor antibody is elevated)
   b. Tests to exclude collagen diseases which are sometimes associated with myasthenia symptom
4. Chest X-ray to exclude respiratory infection and carcination or thymic tumor.
5. Electromyography: EMG differentiates between presynaptic and postsynaptic defects and can identify the defect at the myoneural junction.
6. A complete body scan.

Management Consists of Two Groups of Drugs

1. *Anticholinesterase drugs:*
   a. Neostigmine (prostigmine) 0.5 to 1 mg x 6th hourly (IM) in case of severe weakness. It enhances cholinergic action by facilitating the transmission of impulses across the neuromuscular function. As a parasympathetic stimulant it inhibits the destruction of acetylcholine by cholinesterase thus enhancing the transmission of impulses across the myoneural junction.
   b. It starts to act within 20 minutes and its peak effect occurs within about 2 ½ hours.
   c. Atropine is the antidote for anticholinesterase drugs. Must be available for any patients receiving anticholinesterase therapy.
2. *Pyridostigmine (Mestinon):* as oral dose. It also inhibits the destruction of cholinesterase. The dosage is approximately 60 to 180 mg tds. Action is longer and smoother than neostigmine. 60 mg q 6th hourly.
3. *Immunomodulation:* Prednisolone—corticosteroids (1 mg/kg) and/or azathioprime 3 mg/kg (is given in long standing problems). The usual precautions of steroid therapy, giving potassium supplement, tapering dosage and giving antacids should be followed.
4. *Thymectomy:* Thymectomy for hyperplasia which is apparently in 80 percent of patients are recommended. The procedure induces a remission of symptoms in approximately 40 percent of patients.
5. *Plasmapheresis:* It is a process of washing acetylcholine receptor antibodies which interfere with normal function of acetylcholine receptor sites, from the plasma. The procedure takes 3 to 5 hours. The plasma exchange is done at the bed side with a blood cell separator machine. Albumin is used as plasma exchanger. The plasma exchange is done every alternate day. An improvement in muscle strength is noted about 24 to 48 hours after first exchange.

Myasthenic Crisis versus Cholinergic Crisis

Myasthenic crisis: It is a sudden exacerbation of myasthenic symptom. May occur due to infection or any other reason. The symptoms may be difficulty with swallowing, breathing, finally respiratory failure.

Cholinergic crisis: Occurs due to toxic levels of anticholinesterase drugs. May develop muscarinic and nicotinic effects described earlier. Patient may have abdominal cramping and diarrhea, later generalized weakness, excessive pulmonary secretions and impaired respiratory function.

The tensilon test is used to differentiate myasthenic crisis from cholinergic crisis. An improvement in muscle strength upon injection of the drug suggest the diagnosis of myasthenic crisis.

Management of both crises requires intubation and ventilatory support. Monitoring vital capacity and blood gas levels and needs intensive medical and nursing management.

Nursing Care of Myasthenia Gravis

Myasthenia patients are hospitalized for evaluation and diagnosis, during myasthenic or cholinergic crisis, during intermittent infection with pneumonia or for the thymectomy.

When they are admitted with acute problems they usually have respiratory problems and swallowing difficulties. During this period, they will be placed in intensive care unit for constant monitoring. Ventilatory assistance may be provided or sometime they may need tracheostomy to alleviate respiratory problems.

General Care

1. *Assess the degree of strength or weakness:* Of all muscle involved (respiratory, voice, hand grasp, leg movement and extraocular muscles).
   - Note the time of day when patient is weakest and inform the physician so that drug adjustment can be done accordingly.
   - Help the patient to plan his daily schedule, so that sufficient rest is provided during the activities.
   - Encourage the patient to identify stressors and adjust life-style to decrease the peaks of high physical activities.
2. *Observe for respiratory problems:* If so, take definite action to support an adequate breathing pattern.
3. *Eating and drinking:* Patient will have difficulty in chewing and swallowing:
   - Ryles tube feeding is preferred most of the time.
   - If patient is on oral diet, observe for aspiration and teach the technique of preventing aspiration.

- Tab Tyridostigmine to be given 30 to 45 mts before meal time.
- Soft high protein diet is encouraged in the form of minced or pured.

4. *Elimination:* Very occasionally patient may have incontinence of urine due to weakness of pelvic floor muscles which is transitory, understanding the patient problem will reduce the patient embarrassment.
   - Constipation is not usually a feature in this case. But enema should never be given as it may precipitate crisis.
5. *Personal hygiene:*
   - Patient may need some assistance in maintaining their personal hygiene.
   - Hot baths and sun baths should be avoided as they tend to exacerbate the symptoms.
6. *Psychological support:*
7. *Patient teaching*: Patients with myasthenia gravis are usually managed at home. The more the patient knows about the disease and the treatment, the less likely is a patient to develop complication.
   - Patient and relatives to be taught about the illness and how to adopt his/her lifestyle to live with the problem.
   - They should be made familiar with the drugs as well as the side effects of the drug; and the possible crisis and the treatment to be given.
   - An ambubag and portable suction device should be made available at home for patient who are prone to crisis.
   - Patient teaching also should include
     - To have identity card indicating his disease and dosage of drug taken, etc.
     - To take medicine 30 minutes before meal.
     - To eat slowly and to select soft diet.
     - To avoid infections, extreme temperature, exposure to sun.
     - To provide adequate rest periods during day.
     - Set priorities and plan ahead so that undue fatigue is avoided.
     - Wear sensible shoes to minimize weakness and loss of balance.
     - To avoid emotional stress.

PLASMAPHERESIS (PLASMA EXCHANGE)

Pheresis means separation. Plasmapheresis is a therapeutic procedure where plasma containing antibodies/pathological substance is separated from the blood and remaining components of blood is returned back to the patient. It is performed for patients suffering from autoimmune disorders like:

1. Guillain-Barré syndrome
2. Myasthenia gravis
3. Polymyositis
4. Multiple sclerosis
5. Autoimmune vasculitis
6. Chronic inflammatory demyelinating disorders
7. Acute inflammatory demyelinating polyradiculopathy

   It also done in other non-neurological autoimmune disorders like
   - Thrombotic thrombocytopenic purpura
   - Systemic lupus erythromatus SLE, etc.

Purpose of the procedure: It is a nonspecific treatment. The purpose is to remove antibodies, antigen antibody complexes and mediators of inflammation present in the blood, which are responsible for tissue damage, so that the attack to target tissue or organ is diminished. It brings significant improvement in patient's symptoms.

Plasmapheresis done in two ways:

1. Small volume PP.
2. Large volume PP.

Small Volume PP (Semiautomatic)

- Here the team identifies the patient as per the request from the clinicians.
- After a medical examination and assessing the fitness, Phlebotomy is done and about 450 ml of blood, in adults is collected and IV saline is given to the patient. In children and under-weight adults 11 ml/kg blood is collected.
- The blood is centrifuged at 4000/rpm for 9 minutes and plasma is removed without disturbing the layers in the blood bag. The plasma is weighed and discarded. Equal amount of (plasma weight) normal saline is mixed with the cells and infused into the blood bag and sent to the patient for transfusion.

After infusing cells FFP (fresh frozen plasma) is infused in equal quantity of plasma removed.

Large Volume Plasmapheresis (Automatic)

The indication for large volume plasmapheresis is the same as that of small volume plasmapheresis. But patient with severe illness is preferred in order to avoid patient developing respiratory distress or bulbar symptoms.

The procedure is done at transfusion medicine center in plasmapheresis room. After thorough examination of the patient for fitness to undergo plasmapheresis, patient is made to lie on the couch. The needle is inserted into one of the antecubital vein and the flow of blood is adjusted. On the other arm IV line is started to infuse hematocele or expand. Plasmapheresis is done using the cell separator. The cell separator used is intermittent type. That means in the same arm blood is drawn and cells, after separation of plasma is reinfused. The amount of extracorporeal blood should not exceed 13 percent of total blood volume. The amount of plasma pheresed and amount of colloid (hematocele) infused are balanced.

After the procedure patient is sent to the ward and instructed not to walk for next 6 hours (if the patient is ambulatory). Fresh frozen plasma (FFP) is infused in the ward. The amount of FFP to be infused depends upon the amount of plasmapheresed. As a replacement solution albumin preparation can also be used if the patient is affordable. The albumin solution will cost about 10 to 15 thousands. Whereas FFP is about 200 to 300 rupees. This is non-specific, time-consuming, costly and risky procedure. It requires constant monitoring of the patient during the procedure. Even after the procedure patient should be watched for minimum of 6 hours.

Nurses' Responsibility

1. Proper and clear information to be given about the purpose and technique of the procedure.
2. Collecting blood from the patient and after processing sending it back to the patient with proper labeling.
3. Monitoring patient vital signs during plasmapheresis.
4. Administering IV fluids. After removing the blood and FFP after infusing cells back to patient.
5. Being a team member do supporting team activity.

18

Cranial Nerve Disorders

TRIGEMINAL NEURALGIA (FIG. 18.1)

Trigeminal neuralgia (tic Douloureux) is a disease affecting fifth cranial nerve, characterized by intense paroxysmal pain in the distribution of one or more branches of the trigeminal nerve.

Clinical Presentation

1. Pain is abrupt in onset, unilateral and lasts for a few seconds to a few minutes.
2. Pain is described as paroxysmal, sharp, piercing, shooting, burning and lightning in nature.
3. No motor or sensory deficit is found.
4. Frequency of pain ranges from several times daily to once or twice a month.
5. Patient may describe a trigger that induces the paroxysms, e.g. chewing, facial movements or light touch. Patients may avoid talking, eating or to attend personal hygiene such as washing face, brushing for fear of precipitating pain.

Causes

Causes unknown. But suggested causes are

1. Degenerative or fibrotic changes in the gasserian ganglion
2. Compression of trigeminal nerve by a tumor or a blood vessel or aneurysm.

Diagnosis

1. History and observations
2. Stimulation of triggering points.

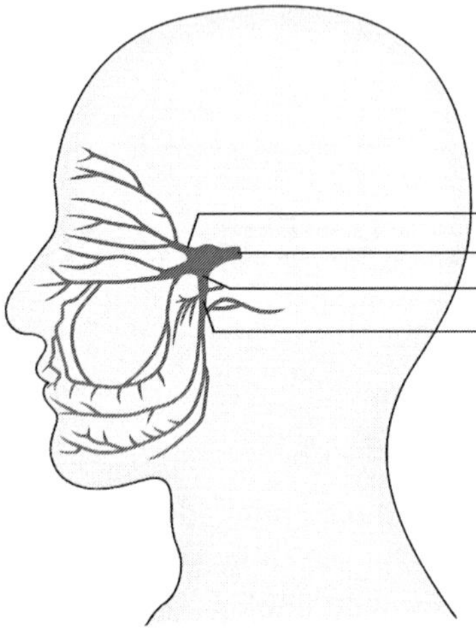

Fig. 18.1: Trigeminal neuralgia

Anatomy

The trigeminal nerve emerges from the pons passing across the Petrous ridge to become gasserian ganglion, which in turn separates into the ophthalmic, maxillary and mandibular division. It is the largest of the cranial nerves possessing both motor and sensory components.

Course

Patient may experience bouts of pain for several weeks or months followed by spontaneous remission. Remission varies from days to years.

Treatment

1. Commonly used drugs are:
   i. Carbomazepine (Tegretol) 200 mg 2 to 5 times a day. It induces remissions in a high percentage of patients.
   ii. Phenytoin.
   iii. Baclofen 40 mg/day.
2. Alcohol or phenol block:
   i. Injection of alcohol or phenol into one or more branches of trigeminal nerve or directly into the ganglion is done. Relief of

pain lasts for 8 to 16 months. Complete blocking of gasserian ganglion may cause complete anesthesia to a portion of the face.

3. Surgery:
   i. Radiofrequency selective thermal rhizotomy of the trigeminal ganglion or rootlets can be performed percutaneously with local anesthesia in conjunction with short-acting barbiturates. Selective distraction of pain fibers is done.
   ii. Microvascular decompression of trigeminal nerve—An intracranial approach to decompress (remove pressure from) trigeminal nerve.
   iii. Open surgical retrogasserian rhizotomy—Destruction of retrogasserian rootlets.

Nursing Care

1. Recognize that certain factors may aggravate excruciating pain.
2. Assist the patient to identify those activities that trigger pain and plan strategies to control the precipitating factors.
3. Administer pain medication at the first indication of paroxysmal bouts of pain.
4. Encourage the patient to take care of personal hygiene between bouts of pain.
5. Instruct the patient to:
   a. Take foods and fluids at room temperature.
   b. Chew soft foods on unaffected side.
   c. Rinse mouth with room temperature water after eating if tooth brushing precipitates pain.
   d. Use cotton pads with room temperature water to wash face
   e. To maintain a written weekly record of weight.
6. Patient will have anxiety, depression and insomnia because of chronic painful condition. Plan appropriate nursing care and referrals if needed.

   Following surgical interventions, instruct the patient:
   a. To instill artificial tears in eyes every 4 hours if there is a marked loss of corneal sensation.
   b. To chew on unaffected side of mouth until accustomed to numbness. Avoid biting lips, tongue or inside of mouth.
   c. To do jaw opening exercises as directed.
   d. To visit a dental doctor for regular check-up.

FACIAL PARALYSIS OR BELL'S PALSY (FIG. 18.2)

Facial paralysis or Bell's palsy is an acute paralysis of 7th cranial nerve producing weakness or paralysis of one side of the facial muscle.

Etiology is unknown:

1. The possible causes are
   a. Viral infection
   b. Idiopathic
   c. Granulomatous disease, e.g. sarcoidosis
   d. Autoimmune disease or a combination of these three.

Majority of patients have a viral prodrome upper respiratory infection 1 to 3 weeks before onset of symptoms.

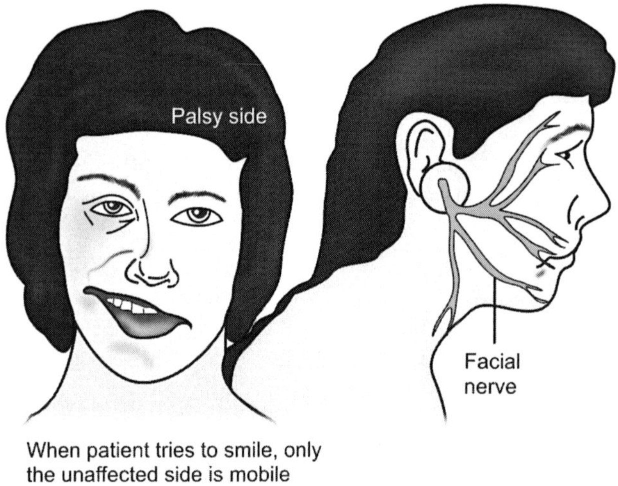

Fig. 18.2: While smiling only the unaffected side moves

Signs and Symptoms

1. Bell's palsy may be preceded by symptoms of pain behind the ear, or on the face for a few hour or days prior to the onset.
2. Drawing sensation on the affected side of the face followed by paralysis of facial muscles.
3. Facial numbness, diminished taste and numbness of tongue.
4. Painful sensation in face, behind ear and in the eye.
5. Eyes do not close and the forehead does not wrinkle.
6. Patient cannot smile, whistle or grimace.

7. The affected side of the face is mask like and sags.
8. Constant tearing and drooling may be present.
9. Speech difficulties may be present.

Diagnosis

1. History and clinical examination
2. Test of cranial function and corneal sensation
3. Electrophysiologic testing.

Course and Prognosis

1. It occurs at any age but most frequently between 20 to 60 years.
2. Eighty percent will recover completely within a few weeks or a few months.

Treatment

1. Tab Prednisone 80 mg per oral daily for 5 days followed by a 7 days taper dosage.
2. Analgesics are given for pain.
3. Massage, moist heat, electrical stimulation with the nerve may be given.
4. When the muscle tone improves, grimacing, wrinkling the brow, whistling and blowing air out should be practised daily for 5 minutes in front of the mirror.

Complications

- Corneal ulceration
- Impairment of vision
- Corneal perforation.

Nursing Care

1. Reassure the patient that he is not having the stroke and recovery will probably occur completely.
2. Protect the involved eye as blinking reflex is absent.
3. Prevent the drying of cornea to avoid corneal ulcers.
   a. Keep the cornea moist with artificial tears instilled into affected eye at regular intervals
   b. Close eyelids periodically

   c. Increase environmental humidity to keep the cornea moist
   d. Avoid drying from sun, wind or air conditioning
   e. Avoid eye irritants, such as fumes, cosmetics.
4. Ensure eye protection during sleep
   a. Use eye ointment at bed time.
   b. Tape upper lid closed by a strip of ¼ inch paper tape fixed to the skin.
   c. Report eye pain immediately.
5. Continue to use facial massage to maintain muscle tone.
6. Keep the face warm and free from draught.
7. Provide frequent small feedings of soft food as patient will have problems in chewing, swallowing and control of saliva on the affected side.
8. Teach the patient the following exercises to do in front of the mirror:
   a. Raise eyebrows
   b. Squeeze eyes closed
   c. Purse the lips
   d. Move mouth from side to side
   e. Blow out cheeks, smile
   f. Whistle.
9. Provide psychological and emotional support to cope with radical change in self concept and body image.

MÉNIÈRE'S DISEASE

Ménière's disease is the disorder of VIII cranial nerve involving both vestibular and cochlear branches. It is thought to be the result of fluid accumulation in the endolymphatic space.

Symptoms

1. Sudden attacks of vertigo are often severe enough to fling the person to the ground.
2. Attacks last few minutes to several hours and patient may vomit repeatedly.
3. Tinnitus develops in one ear gradually increases deafness.
4. Nystagmus and unsteadiness will be present during the attack.
5. The attacks vary in frequency and severity with remissions in between.
6. Eventually the vertigo stops leaving severe deafness.

7. Pain is usually unilateral, 10 percent patients have bilateral.
8. Both sexes are affected, fifth decade is the most frequent time of the onset.

Diagnosis

1. History and clinical findings
2. Caloric test and audiometry.

Treatment

During the attack
1. Bedrest
2. Encourage to try different recumbent positions until one that minimizes the vertigo
3. Salt restricted diet
4. Drugs: Vasodilator and diuretics are given, sometimes sedatives are given.

Tab. Diamox 1 bd (reduces formation of endolymph)

Acute attack – Injection Stemetil 1 amp/Injection calmpose IV
– Complete bedrest
– Positional exercise of head to reduce vertigo

Vestibular sedatives are: – Tab Dilligan
– Avomin
– Stemetil
– Stuzoron 5 mg tds or bd.

Surgery

1. Labyrinthin destruction is done for the patients with unilateral disease where complete deafness will occur.
2. In bilateral disease the vestibular portion of 8th nerve is resected intracranially or the labyrinth is resected selectively with cryotherapy.

Nursing Care

1. Prevent accident from falling.
2. Provide emotional support throughout illness.

As the condition may prolong with repeated attacks for a long time emotional support to be continuous and strength providing. Patient should be instructed to carry most effective sedatives or pain relievers always with him/her.

19

Peripheral Neuropathy

Peripheral nervous system can be defined as part of the nervous system that lies outside the pia-arachnoid membrane and is in relation with Schwann cells. This peripheral nervous system is made up of spinal roots, ganglia, peripheral nerves and all cranial nerves except optic and olfactory nerves. It has three components viz. motor, sensory and autonomic subserve the function of motion, sensation and homeostasis.

Peripheral neuropathies are caused by deranged function and structure of peripheral motor, sensory and autonomic neurons.

Epidemiology

Bradley (1981) estimated total incidence of peripheral neuropathy is an industrialized society to be at least 50 per 100,000 per year. Peripheral neuropathy constituted 8.5 and 7 per 1000 hospital admissions from North West India (Kaur *et al* 1982).

Pathological Changes

In general the pathological reactions can be divided into four main categories.

1. Wallerian degeneration which is the response to axonal interruption.
2. Axonal degeneration or axonopathy.
3. Primary neuronal (perikaryal) degeneration or neuronopathy.
4. Segmental degeneration.

Patient's signs and symptoms and characteristics of nerve conduction study provide information about the underlying pathological changes.

Wallerian degeneration: Any type of mechanical injuries can cause interruption of axon, leading to Wallerian degeneration (degeneration of axons and their myelin sheath) distal to the site of transection.

Motor weakness and sensory loss are immediate in the distribution of damaged nerve. The proximal end of distal stump becomes swollen and myelin retracts from axons, beginning at the nodes of Ranvier. On the third day, the axon becomes shrunken later fragments.

The quality of recovery depends on the degree of preservation of Schwann cells—basal lamina tube and the nerve sheath and surrounding tissue and the age of the individual.

Axonal degeneration: This is the most common pathological reaction of peripheral nerve. Presumably caused by metabolic derangement within the neurons. The myelin sheath breaks down concomitantly with the axon in a process that starts at the most distal part of the nerve fiber and progress toward the nerve cell body hence the term dying back neuropathy. It presents with symmetrical, distal loss of sensory and motor functions in the lower extremities and extend proximally in a graded manner.

Axonal regeneration proceeds at a rate of 2 to 3 mm per day, recovery may be delayed and is often incomplete.

Neuronopathy: Designates primary loss on destruction of nerve cell bodies with resultant degeneration of entire peripheral and central axons. Either lower motor neurons or dorsal root ganglion cells may be affected.

Segmental demyelination: Implies injury of myelin sheath or Schwann cells; resulting in breakdown of myelin sheath with sparing of axons. This occurs in immune mediated demyelinating neuropathies and in heriditary disorders of Schwann cells.

Myelin metabolism: A part or whole segment is damaged during demyelination. Here the recovery begins early and is often complete. Proximal weakness is more prominent.

The functional consequence of demyelination is conduction block resulting in motor weakness and mild sensory loss. Recovery depends on remyelination which is relatively fast and clinical improvement may occur within days to weeks. Axonal degeneration and segmental degeneration coexist in neuropathies.

Course

Neuropathy may be:

1. Acute—less than four weeks
2. Subacute—four weeks to eight weeks
3. Chronic—more than eight weeks

Relapsing course is observed in chronic relapsing inflammatory demyelinating neuropathy.

Causes of Neuropathies

1. Infections
   a. Leprosy
   b. Inflammation or demyelination
      i. G.B. syndrome
      ii. Diphtheritic neuropathy
2. Genetic disorders
   a. Familial amyloidosis
   b. Porphyria
   c. Leukodystrophies
   d. Fabry's disease, etc.
3. Poisons: (metals, drugs and industrial chemicals)
   a. Arsenic neuropathy
   b. Lead neuropathy
   c. Drugs
      i. INH
      ii. Nitrofurantoin
      iii. Vincristine
      iv. Chloramphenicol
      v. Organophosphates—triorthocresylphosphate (TCP), used as plastic softner and lubricant.
         —Suicidal attempt with insecticides (TEPP)
4. Nutritional neuropathy
   a. Alcoholic neuropathy due to B-complex deficiency
5. Metabolic causes
   a. Diabetes
   b. Uremia
   c. Porphyria
   d. Amyloidosis
6. Endocrine disorders
   a. Acromegaly
   b. Hypothyroidism
   c. Carcinoma
   d. Lymphoma
7. Vascular
   a. Increased BP
   b. Collagen diseases

8. Mechanical trauma
   a. Trauma
   b. Compression.

Signs and Symptoms

- Patients may experience tingling, pricking, burning sensation, and like dysthesia in the balls of the feet or tips of the toes
- Symmetry of the symptoms
- Sensory loss in a graded stocking fashion
- Weakness
- Numbness or wooden feeling—patient may say I feel as though I am walking on a stump
- Unsteady gait
- Muscle atrophy
- Difficulty walking during night
- Piano playing fingers
- Locomotor ataxia
- Muscle cramps and fasciculations
- Dysthesia—unpleasant, abnormal sensation in response to an ordinary painless stimulus
- *Paresthesia:* An unpleasant sensation arising spontaneously allodynia or hyperpathia—perception of nonpainful stimuli as painful
- Paresthesia
- Neuropathic pain often has a deep burning character that may be associated with jobbing or shooting pains and typically increases at periods of rest.

Diagnosis

Diagnosis done by
- History
- Blood, urea/glucose
- Liver function test
- VDRL
- Collagen
- Peripheral smear
- GTT
- ENMG

Types of Neuropathies

In neuropathy the deficit may be of a single nerve—mononeuropathy.

Multiple individual nerves are involved—mononeuropathy multiplex.

Diffuse bilateral involvement—polyneuropathy.

Neuropathy may be purely motor, sensory, autonomic or mixed. Mixed polyneuropathy is the most common form.

The following are the conditions seen in different neuropathies

a. Predominantly motor neuropathy is seen in
    i. Guillain-Barré syndrome
    ii. Porphyria
    iii. Diphtheria
    iv. Hereditary motor sensory neuropathy
    v. Hypoglycemia
    vi. Depsone toxicity
    vii. Lead poison.
b. Pure sensory neuropathy is seen in
    i. Diabetes mellitus
    ii. Carcinoma
    iii. Amyloidosis, etc.
c. Autonomic dysfunction can be prominent feature in
    i. Guillain-Barré syndrome
    ii. Diabetes mellitus
    iii. Alcoholic neuropathy
    iv. Porphyria and familial dysautonomia.

Mononeuropathy is where one nerve is affected commonly due to trauma, external pressure or bad positioning, etc.

The causes are:

a. Trauma: Mechanical, thermal, electrical
b. Entrapment and compression
c. Infections: Herpes zoster, leprosy, syphilis
d. Vascular: Necrotising angiopathy, peripheral vascular disease, embolism, hemorrhage
e. Toxins: Vaccines, lead
f. Infiltration: Tumors, sarcoidosis.

This neuropathy may be acute or chronic. The nerves affected may be

- Median nerve (Carpal tunnel syndrome)
- Ulnar nerve

- Sciatic nerve
- Femoral nerve
- Tibial nerve
- Common peroneal nerve, etc.

Mononeuropathy Multiplex

Most of the lesions listed for mononeuropathies can also produce focal lesions of multiple nerves.
The more frequent causes include

- Leprosy
- Diabetes mellitus
- Necrotising angiopathy
- Amyloidosis
- Acquired inflammatory demyelinating neuropathy.

Inflammatory Demyelinating Polyradiculoneuropathies

Inflammatory demyelinating polyradiculoneuropathies are acquired immune mediated neuropathies. It is classified into acute inflammatory demyelinating polyradiculopathy (AIDP) and chronic inflammatory demyelinating polyradiculopathy (CIDP) by their clinical course. AIDP is also termed as Guillain-Barré syndrome which is discussed in detail in a different chapter of this book.

Chronic Inflammatory Demyelinating Polyradiculoneuropathy (CIDP)

Acute inflammatory demyelinating polyradiculopathy (AIDP) and CIDP are similar except for the time course. Most CIDP patients have a continuous or stepcoire progressive course over months to years, but one-third have a relapsing course with partial or complete recovery between recurrences.

Clinical Features

- Peak incidence is in fifth and sixth decades
- Weakness more than 2 months period
- All limbs are affected, the legs more severely

- Numbness or tingling (but not pain) are experienced in a stocking glove distribution
- Symmetric motor sensory neuropathy with both proximal and distal involvement
- Large fibers are affected more frequently and severely
- Involvement of trunk muscle is uncommon and of cranial nerves infrequent.

Diagnosis

- CSF studies
- Nerve biopsy
- NCV changes.

Treatment

- Prednisone 1 to 1.5 mg per kg per day started as single dose, tapered after 4 weeks. Over 3 to 4 months to maintenance dose of 20 to 40 mg per day.
- Plasma exchange
- Intravenous immunoglobulin are beneficial—2 gm per day 3 days.

Nursing Care

As discussed in Guillain-Barré syndrome (AIDP).

General Nursing Care of Patient with Peripheral Neuropathy

- Take detail history of illness, do all the neurochemical investigations looking for any deficiency and treat accordingly.
- The nursing care consists of relieving the symptoms and providing comfortable measures like covering the extremities while resting, providing supportive measures like use of crape bandages, etc.
- When patient is having loss of sensation or no sensation in the part, the nursing care should be directed towards to prevent injuries. The measures to be taken are:
    i. Advice not to handle hot water and hot foods
    ii. Avoid working near the fire
    iii. Special precautions to be taken while they work with sharp instruments and machinery

iv. Ladies working in the kitchen should use the sharp instruments very carefully.

- Care of foot is extremely important in patients with peripheral neuropathy.
    i. They should be advised to use footwear all the time.
    ii. Footwear should be proper fitting and should not have nails.
    iii. Foot should be washed with warm salt water everyday, giving attention in between the toes.
    iv. The feet should be checked for cracks and cuts everyday so that immediate care can be given.
- Family and patient should be explained about the progress of the disease and appropriate measures should be adopted in rehabilitation of the patient.

20

Wilson's Disease (Hepatolenticular Degeneration)

Wilson's disease is an autosomal recessive error in copper metabolism that is associated with hepatic cirrhosis and degenerative changes in the basal ganglia.

Etiology

- This is a rare inherited disorder carried by an autosomal recessive gene
- Affects children of both sexes if both parents are carriers
- The disorder is due to abnormal copper metabolism.

Pathology

Daily dietary intake of copper ranges between 2 to 5 mg/day. Normally copper ingested in certain food stuffs in the diet is absorbed in small amount through the gut, loosely bound to albumin, and carried to the liver, where most of it is excreted in the bile. A small about becomes firmly bound to globulin, forming ceruloplasmin (copper transport protein) in the blood.

In Wilson's disease excessive amounts of copper are absorbed through gut, the bonding with globulin is defective (therefore the ceruloplasm level is low) and copper is free. Much of it is excreted in the urine. But a smaller, damaging proportion is deposited in the liver, brain, kidney tubules, basal ganglia and the membrane lining the posterior surface of the cornea (Descemet's membrane). Pathologically, there are postneurotic cirrhosis of the liver, degeneration of the renal tubular epithelial cells, spongy degeneration of the basal ganglia with large numbers of protoplasmic astrocytes and granular clumping of copper in the endothelial surface of Descemet's membrane of cornea.

Signs and Symptoms

- Patients may present with rapid onset of hepatic failure in early childhood.
- Neurologic manifestation begins around the age 10 to 12 years.
- Patients will have slow progressive dysarthria and dysphagia.
- Tremor and rigidity similar to Parkinsonism.
- Characteristic dystonic grim with a mask like face and bradykinesia.
- Excessive salivation and drooling.
- Emotional lability.
- Progressive intellectual deterioration and dementia.

Diagnosis

1. Diagnosis is supported by the finding of copper storage in the cornea on slit lamp examination (Kayser-Fleischer ring).
2. Test related to copper metabolism
   - serum copper estimation
   - ceruloplasmin estimation
   - 24-hour collection of urine for copper excretion
3. Liver function test
4. Renal function test
5. Psychometry.

Treatment

1. Without treatment Wilson's disease is fatal within few years.
2. Most effective drug is oral penicillamine, a chelating agent, which absorbs copper from the liver, brain and kidneys and aids its excretion in the urine.
3. Penicillamine 250 mg 3 to 4 times a day before meals and continued for the rest of the patient's life.
4. Zincap 1 tds
5. Ferrous sulphate daily
6. Regular blood and urine tests should be performed throughout treatment to determine copper levels and detect any adverse changes in blood picture. (Penicillamine causes bone marrow suppression and glomerular nephritis).

Nursing Care

As there is no cure for the patients with Wilson's disease, care can be only symptomatic, prevention of complications, psychological support to patient and family members. Few points to be remembered while nursing these patients are:

- Protect the patient from fall.
- Avoid foods which are rich in copper, e.g. shellfish, liver, mushroom, broccoli cereals, chocolate and nuts.
- Should be given good nutrition to prevent other nutritional disorders and general infection.
- Educate the patient and family about the need for life long treatment.
- Patient should be explained the progress of the disease and to live with the disability.
- Patient can be referred to other organizations to get financial and other supports.

21

Myopathies

Definition

Myopathies means primary structural or functional impairment of muscles.

Classifications

Myopathies can be classified as hereditary and acquired disorders.

1. Hereditary disorders can be classified:
   - Muscular dystrophies
   - Congenital myopathies
   - Myotonias channelopathies
   - Metabolic myopathies
   - Mitochondrial myopathies
2. Acquired disorders are classified as:
   - Inflammatory
   - Endocrine myopathies
   - Myopathies associated with systemic illness
   - Drug induced/toxic myopathies.

Hereditary Disorders

a. Muscular dystrophies
   There are various kinds of muscular dystrophies, like congenital muscular dystrophy, fascioscapulohumeral dystrophy, limb-girdle muscular dystrophy, etc. These are discussed in separate chapter (muscular dystrophies) in this book.

b. Congenital myopathies
   Deformities due to shortening and fibrosis of muscles, examples
   - Clubfoot
   - Congenital elevation of scapula
   - Talipes equinovarus
   - Dorsiflexion of feet and ankle

Congenital wryneck begins during the first month of life and is due to shortening of the sternomastoid muscle.

Nemalline myopathy is the hypotonia and impaired motility in infancy and early childhood.

c. Myotonia channelopathies

It is the phenomenon of impaired relaxation of muscle after forceful voluntary contraction.

d. Metabolic myopathies
   - Glycogen storage diseases
   - Lipid storage myopathies
   - Familial periodic paralysis
     Hypokalemic
     Normokalemic
     Hyperkalemic
   - Alcoholic myopathies
   - Protein deficiency—Kwashiorkor
     —Malabsorption
   - Calcium metabolism related
   - Osteomalacia
   - Nutritional deficiency
   - Anticonvulsants
   - Malabsorption
   - Wilson's disease

e. Mitochondrial myopathies

It is an abnormal accumulation of lipid bodies in muscle fibers.
   - When large number of mitochondria accumulation occurs in the cell is called "plesconial myopathies."
   - When giant type of mitochondria accumulation occurs in the cell, then it is called "megaconial myopathies."

Acquired Myopathies

a. Inflammatory

Inflammatory myopathies are polymyositis, dermatomyositis, (discussed in separate chapter).

b. Endocrine myopathies
   - Thyroid
   - Hyperthyroid myopathies
   - Myasthenia gravis
   - Periodic paralysis
   - Hypothyroid myopathy

- Pituitary
- Hypopituitarism
- Acromegaly with muscle hypertrophy
- Cushing's disease
- Adrenal
- Addison's disease

c. Myopathies associated with systemic illness
Myopathies associated with other diseases as cardiac disease, peripheral vascular disease, hepatomegaly.

d. Drug induced myopathy
Sometimes myopathies occur due to chronic use of the following drugs
- Steroids
- Chloroquin
- Emetine
- Vincristine
- Pentazocin, etc.

e. Toxic myopathies
Sometimes alcoholism may cause proximal muscle weakness. After snake bites also myopathies occurs.

Signs and Symptoms

- Weakness of the muscles
- Weakness in the legs
- Difficulty in climbing stairs, rising from the low chair toilet or floor
- Ankle weakness due to distal muscle weakness
- Dysarthria
- Dysphagia
- Drooping eyelids.

Diagnostic Procedure is done by

- History
- Symptoms
- Neurological examination.

Investigations

- Serum enzymes of muscle—creatinine kinase (CK) occurs in high concentration in the ceruloplasmin of skeletal and cardiac muscle.

- EMG is done at rest and at activity
- Muscle biopsy
- Urine analysis.

Treatment

a. Medical
b. Nursing.

Medical

- No specific treatment.
- Sometimes quinine has a mild action at the motor end plate and thus relieves myotonia—Dose - 0.3 gm to 0.6 gm orally bd.
- Procanamide, phenytoin, ACTH and corticosteroids are sometime useful in alleviating, myotonia.

Nursing

- Avoid prolonged bedrest.
- To encourage the patient to maintain as full and normal life as possible.
- Muscular dystrophy—persons encouraged for any sedentary occupation.

Prognosis

- If the disease is acute, patient may have remissions. But, if the patient suffers for long-time, then muscle disability may occur.

Complications

- Pulmonary or cardiac complications
- Weakness of the hip and shoulder
- Disability in normal life.

INFLAMMATORY MYOPATHIES

Inflammatory myopathy may occur either due to:

1. Infection
    - Virus

      The most common viruses that affect the muscles are
      - Coxsackie

  - Herpes simplex
  - Influenza
  - HIV
- Bacteria—staphylococcal
- Parasites
  - Toxoplasma
  - Cysticercosis
  - Trichinosis

2. Autoimmune myopathies are of various types like polymyositis (PM) and dermatomyositis (DM).

The myopathies may be localized like focal nodular, monomelic, orbital or associated with linear scleroderma or panniculitis.

POLYMYOSITIS

Polymyositis means weakness of all muscles. It was first described in 1863.

Definition

Polymyositis is a subacute symmetric weakness of proximal limbs and trunk muscles without dermatitis or with minimal skin lesions.

Etiology

- Unknown.
- Probably it has been used to include disease of viral origin, muscle dystrophies with a few infiltration of inflammatory cells.
- Under electromicroscope it is observed that two types of virus particles are present in the muscle fibers.
- A cellular type of autoimmune reaction is responsible for the muscle fiber neurosis.

Occurrence

- It can occur at any age but common around the ages between 40 to 70 years
- Twenty percent of cases below the age of 15 years
- Females predominate after 7th decade
- Presentation may be acute, subacute or chronic.

Pathology

Destruction of segments of muscle fibers and degeneration of muscle fibers occurs in polymyositis. A large proportion of these cells are CD8 cells (cytotoxic cells).

Fiber necrosis ⟶ Inflammation ⟶ Fibrosis

Signs and Symptoms

- Painless, weakness of the proximal limb muscles especially of the hips and thighs and later extend to shoulder girdles.
- Feeling of difficulties in arising from a chair, or squatting position or kneeling position.
- Difficulty in climbing or descending stairs.
- Difficulty in walking.
- Difficulty in pulling an object from a height.
- Combing the hair becomes difficult.
- Weakness of the neck and quadriceps muscles, facial, pharyngeal and laryngeal muscle also affected.
- Wasting of the shoulder and upper limb girdle muscles may be seen chronic cases.
- Hypertrophy of the calves is seen in 5 percent of patients.
- Contractures occur at a late stage.
- Calcinosis is common in childhood DMN (Dermatomyositis) calcium may be deposited at the site of contractures. Non-healing painful ulcers may be observed at the elbows, groins, dorsum of the hands and soles of the feet extruding calcium flakes from the calcium deposits.

  Diagnosis is made by
  - Blood
  - Urine—Creatinine increased
  - EMG—Shows myopathic features with muscle hyper-irritability
  - Muscle biopsy—Shows scattered fiber necrosis and phagocytosis and perivascular cuffing with inflammatory cells.

Treatment

- Prednisolone (steroid)—2 mg/kg initial dose upto 100 mg when improvement is occurred the dose is reduced to 60 mg daily/alternative days, maintained over several weeks.

- Antibiotics
- Cyclophosphamide and methotrexate also used in some cases.

Prognosis

- Prognosis is better in those patients where adequate therapy has been instituted within 2 months.
- In general, prognosis is not good when polymyositis (PM) is acute or is associated with connective tissue disorders or malignancy.

Nursing Care

Nursing care to be planned according to the signs and symptoms.

DERMATOMYOSITIS

Dermatomyositis occurs in children and adults. It is most common myositis of childhood. In adults it is often associated with an underlying malignancy.

Signs and Symptoms

- Onset of rash may be concurrent or follow the muscle weakness.
- Typical skin rash is seen on the face in a butterfly shape.
- Purplish discoloration of the skin over the cheeks and eyelids on the face in a butterfly shape.
- The weakness is usually proximal more than distal and can be severe.
- Calcinosis is common in childhood DM. Calcium may be deposited at the site of contractures. Nonhealing painful ulcers may be observed at the elbows, groins, dorsum of the hands and soles of the feet extruding calcium flakes from the calcium deposits.
- Muscle pain is sometimes present.
- The illness often follows a relapsing remitting course although occasionally is monophagic to the point of recovering spontaneously without treatment.

Treatment and Nursing Care

Principles of treatment and nursing care in dermatomyositis are the same as for polymyositis.

22

Headache/Cephalgia

Cephalgia or headache is one of the common physical complaint in all age group and in both sexes.

Definition

Headache is defined as occurrence of pain or discomfort over the upper part of head from the orbit to the suboccipital area arising from pain sensitive areas. The skull and the brain are not capable of feeling pain. It is from the scalp muscles and blood vessels and from dura and its venous sinuses that pain is felt.

Headache can be categorized as primary or secondary headache.

Primary headache is a headache for which no organic cause can be consistently identified.

They are:

1. Migraine headache
2. Cluster headache
3. Tension headache.

Secondary headache is associated with a variety of primary organic etiologies.

Migraine Headache

It is generally believed that symptoms are produced by spasms of vessels inside the skull and the dilatation of vessels outside the skull. The spasm produces a warning sign (aura) and the dilatation produces headache.

Incidence

- Usually starts in youth
- Affects women more than men
- May be hereditary
- People who have lower tolerance to stress develops easily.

Signs and Symptoms

- It is unilateral headache.
- Pain will be throbbing in characters (pulsating).
- Pain can be so severe that person will not be able to do usual activity.
- Vomiting, nausea, and photophobia may be present.
- Pain may last for 4 hours to 3 days.
- Pain may be relieved by lying down in a dark place.
- Some may have aura at the beginning of headache. They see a bright spot at center which gradually increases in size, the edges may be flaring. These are called *teichopsia, fortification* and *spectra*. The aura usually lasts for a few minutes.

Migraine Triggers

- Menstrual cycles
- Mental or physical stress
- Sleep deprivation
- Fatigue
- Alcohol
- Some kind of chocolates triggers migraine.

Diagnosis

History and clinical findings.

Treatment

1. Identification and avoidance of precipitating factors.
2. For mild migraine: Nonsteroidal anti-inflammatory drugs ibuprofen or naproxen are given.
3. Abortive therapy: It is taken as soon as headache starts an attempt to cut short. Ergotamine (vasograin, migranil) is usually given.
4. Migraine prophylaxis: To reduce the frequencies and severity of attacks, the following are given
   - Amitryptyline (Elavil)
   - β-Blockers—propranolol, atenolol
   - Calcium channel blockers—verapamil
   - Cyproheptadine—sodium valproate, may be given as a trial for 3 to 6 months.

Nursing Care

1. Assist the client in identifying the stimuli that precipitates the attacks.
2. Provide dark quiet environment.
3. Administer prescribed drugs.
4. Encourage proper diet, adequate rest, exercise and effective stress management techniques to control stress.
5. Document the type and characteristic of headache.

Tension Headache

Tension headache is the second major category of primary headache.

Headache results from sustained contraction of skeletal muscles in the scalp, face, neck and shoulders (verified by electromyelogram).

Etiology

Common causes are anxiety, emotional tension. May occur where there is faulty position of head, neck and shoulder girdles.

Clinical Features

- Bilateral
- Heavy aching pain
- Occurs at any age
- Starts in the morning, slowly increasing by evening
- No prodromal symptoms.

Diagnosis

Clinical findings and history

Treatment

- Identify the psychopathology
- Antidepressant
- Relaxation technique
- Biofeedback.

Nursing Care

1. Do the detail assessment of pain
2. Talk to the patient and listen to the problem

3. Make the patient to ventilate her/his feelings
4. Mild analgesics if prescribed to be given
5. Teach relaxation technique
6. Proper referral can be done
7. Moist heat may be applied.

Cluster Headache

It is also called histaminic cephalgia. It occurs because of sudden histamine release.

Characteristics

- Severe unilateral burning pain, located around the eye.
- Headache lasts for 15 to 180 minutes.
- Comes in groups or clusters. One to 8 episodes of headache daily lasting up to several weeks to months, followed by a period of remission of months to year.
- Associated with symptoms of tearing, nasal congestion, or rhinorrhea, etc. Can be triggered by alcohol or other vasodilate agents.
- Often comes at night.
- There is no aura.

Etiology

- Sensitivity to histamine
- History of allergies
- Familial

Diagnosis

Clinical findings and history.

Treatment

Eliminate foods which precipitate symptom, supportive care.

- Injection: Sumatryptan
Ergotamine 1 mg bd
Methyl sergide 4 to 9 mg daily

Prophylaxis

- Steroids
- Lithium
- Cyproheptadine
- Periactin 8 to 16 mg daily in divided doses.

Nursing Care

Prepare for self management of these headaches.

SECONDARY HEADACHES

Secondary headache occurs due to some pathology. The reasons may be:

1. Meningitis
2. Trigeminal neuralgia
3. Increased ICP
4. Subarachnoid hemorrhage
5. Low pressure headache—e.g. after lumbar puncture
6. Stroke
7. Cerebral venous thrombosis
8. Benign intracranial hypertension
9. Head trauma
10. Disorders of cranium, neck and others.

For secondary headaches, the cause should be identified and treated.

23

Common Drugs Used in Neuroscience Conditions

The discussion in this chapter is on the drugs used for patients with problems of CNS and the spinal cord. It also gives some important responsibilities of nurses regarding the administration of drugs for neuro patients (Table 23.1).

Nursing is an everchanging field. Standard, safety precautions must be followed always while doing nursing in any field. As new research and clinical experience broaden our knowledge, changes in treatment and drug therapy are obviously necessary. So readers are requested to check the product information currently provided by the manufacturer of each drug to verify the recommended dose, the method and duration of administration. It is the responsibility of the treating physician relying on the experience and knowledge of the patient to determine dosages and duration of the drug therapy. Neither the publisher nor the author of the book assume the responsibility for any untoward incident while or after administering the drugs.

Table 23.1: Common drugs used in neuroscience condition

Name/trade name	*Dosage/route*	*Indication*	*Action*	*Side effects*	*Nursing responsibility*
Acyclovir	Herpes simple × 200 mg 5 times × 5 days Herpes zoster 500 mg 5 times daily × 7 days Prophylaxis 200 mg 4 times daily	Genital herpes simplex. Mucocutaneous herpes simplex. HS encephalitis, keratitis, chickenpox	Antiviral, arrests the viral replication	Headache, nausea, Sweating, fall in BP	Drug should not be given in glaucoma patients with depression, renal impairment.
Albendazole	Adults and children 400 mg as single dose hydatid- 400 mg bd with meals × 28 days Cysticercosis 400 mg od × 30 days	Single or mixed intestinal worm infestation including hydatid disease and cysticercosis	Anthelminthics. It acts probably by blocking glucose uptake in parasites and depletion of its glycogen storage	GI tract disorders	Should not be given in patients with hepatic and renal disease pregnancy and lactation
Aspirin	Oral	Pain, acute or chronic inflammation of bones, osteoarthritis,	Analgesic	Bleeding of the GI tract	To be given after the food, Watch for any signs and symptoms of internal bleeding
Carbamezapine	800-1600 mg/day for adult, 10-30 mg/kg children	Partial seizure, patients with psychopathology trigeminal neuralgia	Membrane stabilization by blocking sodium channels	Blurring of vision diplopia, sedation nausea, anorexia, ataxia, headache, skin rashes, hepatic failure	Look for side effects Regular evaluation of drug level in the blood

Contd...

Contd...

Name/trade name	*Dosage/route*	*Indication*	*Action*	*Side effects*	*Nursing responsibility*
Ciprofloxin	75 mg–orally bd	2nd line of treatment for TB	Antibiotic	Long-term usage can cause deafness	—
Clonazepam (Klonopin)	1-20 mg/day divided into 2-3 times a day	Absence seizures, tourettes syndrome, tics	Benzodiazapine sedative, hypnotic drug	Drowsiness and ataxia	Observe for addiction
Dantrolin sodium (Dantrium)	25 mg qid increased to 100 mg qid–oral-	Neuromalignant syndrome, wheelchair bound paraplegia, spasticity of cerebral origin	Antispastic and acts in neuromalignant syndrome	Generalized weakness, nausea, diarrhea, drowsiness	Observe for general weakness
Diamox (Acetazolamide)	5mg PO twice a day	Pseudotumor cerebri	Diuretic to reduce the CSF volume and intracranial pressure	Paresthesia, tinitis, hearing dysfunction, anorexia, nausea, vomiting, diarrhea, poliurea	• Intake and output chart to be maintained to look for polyurea • Observe for side effects
Diazepam (Valium)	Use PO, IV and IM Dosage varies depending upon individual cases	Seizures, anxiety, alcohol withdrawal	Benzodiazapine, sedative, anti-anxiety agent	Sedation, hypotension Respiratory depression, agitation	• IV to be given very slowly, watching the pulse and respirations • Never take diazepam with any other drugs in the same syringe

Contd...

Contd...

Name/trade name	*Dosage/route*	*Indication*	*Action*	*Side effects*	*Nursing responsibility*
Diclofenic sodium	100-150 mg daily in 2-3 divided doses	Rheumatoid arthritis Osteoarthritis, low back pain, ankylosing spondylitis, acute musculoskeletal disorder, painful inflammatory conditions	Anti-inflammatory action besides analgesic and antipyretic. It is inhibitor of prostaglandin synthesis	Epigastric pain, nausea, diarrhea, tiredness, insomnia, skin rash, itching, retention of fluid	Should not be given to peptic ulcer patients, asthmatic patients, pregnant women and during lactation. Never administer in empty stomach
Ergotamine (Dihydroergotamine)	Tab per orally IV = 1 mg	Migraine	Alpha adrenergic/ serotonin antagonist, cranial vasoconstrictor	Precordial tightness, myalgias, paresthesia, nausea	• The drug is contraindicated in coronary artery disease • Usually given after the administration of Promethazine the antiemetic
Ethambutol	15-25 mg/kg/day – orally	2nd line of treatment for TB	Antituberculosis	Long-term usage can cause deafness	—
Fluconazole/ logicam	400 mg daily 2-12 weeks–oral	Vaginal candida cryptococcal meningitis prevention of fungal infection, in patient with malignancy, AIDS, patients with immunosuppressive drugs	Antifungal action	Nausea, vomiting, abdominal pain, diarrhea, headache, hepatotoxicity	Watch for side effects Not to be given to patients with liver diseases

Contd...

Contd...

Name/trade name	*Dosage/route*	*Indication*	*Action*	*Side effects*	*Nursing responsibility*
Gardinal sodium (Phenobarbitone) (Luminal)	60-240 mg adult dose 3-6 mg/kg/day/ children	Epilepsy, status epilepticus	Anticonvulsant	Sedation, respiratory suppression, hypotention, hyperactivity, rash	- Look for over sedation - Health teaching about drug compliance and regular follow-up
Heparin	20,000 units in 500 ml of dextrose at 20 ml/ hour. (800 units/hour maintenance)-IV	Acute embolic or progressive stroke, transient ischemic attack	Antithrombin effect as in conjection with antithrombin III	Hemorrhage and thrombocytopenia	Daily monitoring of prothrombin time. Observe for bleeding from any orifices. Vital signs to be observed for internal hemorrhage
Imeuran (Azathioprine)	100-200 mg PO/day	Myasthenia gravis	Immunosuppressant	Leukopenia, thrombocytopenia, nausea/vomiting, increased secondary infection	- Blood to be sent for differential count - Observe for signs of infection - Look for nausea and vomiting
Immunoglobulin IV–1g	GBS 0.4 gm/kg IV/ day × 5 days CIDP 0.4 gm/kg IV weekly	GB syndrome chronic inflammatory demyelinating polyneuropathy	Immunosuppressive	Renal failure aseptic meningitis enaphylaxis	Hydrate the patient well to avoid renal toxicity; look for symptoms of anaphylactic stroke

Contd...

Contd...

Name/trade name	*Dosage/route*	*Indication*	*Action*	*Side effects*	*Nursing responsibility*
Isoniazid	5 mg/kg/day adults 15-20 mg/kg/day - oral	1st line treatment for TB	Antituberculosis	Nausea vomiting	Should advice to take continuously
Lanuvudin	150 mg bd Zidovudine 2 mg/kg body weight–oral	HIV infections	Inhibits the key reverse transcriptase enzyme of HIV	—	Not to be given to patients with liver problems
Levodopa carbidopa (Sinemet)	25 mg/100 mg thrice a day tapered as clinically indicated	Parkinson disease	Lavodopa is converted to dopamine in the basal ganglia, carbidopa inhibits dopamine production in the periphery	Dyskinesia, dystonia, chorea, confusion, paranoia	—
Liorasal (Baclofen)	10-20 mg thrice a day PO	Dystonia spasticity of multiple sclerosis	Antispasmodic	Confusion, sedation, increased muscular weakness	- Watch for over sedation - Increased muscular weakness and confusion
Mannitol (Osmitrol)	0.25-1.0 g per kg of 20% solution (20 gm/ 100 mg)–IV	Increased intracranial pressures	Osmotic diuretic	Hypotension, dehydration, hyponatremia, renal damage	- Monitor serum ostomality and electrolyte - Observe for dehydration and hypotension, It given always in 20 mts.

Contd...

Contd...

Name/trade name	*Dosage/route*	*Indication*	*Action*	*Side effects*	*Nursing responsibility*
Methyl predniso-lone (Solu-medrol)	Administered IV Doses varies in individual diseases	Traumatic spinal cord injury, multiple sclerosis, inflammatory optic neuritis, pseudotumor cerebri	Anti-inflammatory/Immunosuppressive agent	Peptic ulcer, sodium and fluid retention, hypertension, hyperglycemia	Watch for infection
Metronidazole	400 mg 8th hourly × 7 days	Amoebiasis Giardiasis Trichomonas vaginitis	Antiprotozoal drug It is also used in Trichomonas, Entamoeba hystolytica	Anorexia, nausea, abdominal cramps, headache, glossitis, dryness of mouth	Not to be given in first trimester of pregnancy
Mobendazole	100 mg bd × 5 days 100 mg for threadworm 200 mg twice × 3 days for tapeworm	Round worm, hookworm, threadworm, tapeworm and mixed infestation	Anthelminthics. It acts by blocking glucose uptake in parasites and depletion of its glycogen storage	Diarrhea, nausea, abdominal pain, allergic reactions, loss of hair	Should not be given in pregnancy and in lactation
Neostigmine	Adult 15-30 mg daily with atropine 0.4 to 1.25 mg given by parental route	Myasthenia gravis	Anticholinesterase, inhibits cholinesterase enzyme which breaks down acetylcholine so that neuromuscular transmission is increased	Salivation, sweating, tracheobronchial secretion, miosis, blurring of vision, nausea, breathlessness, incontinence of urine and stool	Always given parent orally, always administered with atropine, not to be administered in urinary blockage or organic obstruction

Contd...

Contd...

Name/trade name	*Dosage/route*	*Indication*	*Action*	*Side effects*	*Nursing responsibility*
Nimesulide	100 mg bd adults, 5 mg/kg/day for children in two or three divided doses	Rheumatoid arthritis, osteoarthritis, other degenerative joint disorder, musculoskeletal disorders	Nonopioid analgesic	Epigastric pain, heart burn, nausea	Not to be given in peptic ulcer, renal impairment, congestive heart failure, cirrhosis of liver and in pregnancies
Nimodipin	30-60 mg–orally 4th hourly	Stroke, due to vasospasm	Slow calcium channel inhibitor	Hypotension	Frequent observation of blood pressure, before administration BP should be checked
Pariodel (Bromocriptine)	2.5 mg-10 mg thrice a day–oral	Parkinson's disease neuroleptic malignant syndrome	Dopamine agonist	Nausea, headache dizziness, fatigue, vomiting	—
Penicillamine (Cuprimina)	125-1000 mg/day divided into 2-4 times a day	Wilson's disease	Copper chelator	Lupus like rash, leukopenia, thrombocytopenia, epigastric pain nausea/diarrhea	It may precipitate myasthenia gravis—so observe for it
Phenytoin (Dilantin)	200-300 mg as od dose adult 5-6 mg/kg/day od /bd for children	Partial, secondary, generalized seizure	—	Nystagmus, ataxia, gingival, hyperplasia, headache, cardiac arrhythmia	• Look for cardiac arrhythmia

Contd...

Contd...

Name/trade name	*Dosage/route*	*Indication*	*Action*	*Side effects*	*Nursing responsibility*
Praziquantel	Neurocysticercosis 50 mg/kg body weight daily in 3 doses × 15 days *T. solium* and *saginata* 10 mg/kg as single dose	Neurocysticercosis Dermalcysticercosis Intestinal tapeworm infestation	It is rapidly taken up by the susceptible worms and appears to act by causing leakage of intercellular calcium from the membranes leading to contracture and paralysis of worms	GI disorders, abdominal pain, headache, rashes over body	Not to be given in ocular cysticercosis pregnancies and lactation
Prednisone	100 mg orally/day Tapered slowly over several weeks	Temporal arteritis	Anti-inflammatory agent and immunosuppressant	Peptic ulcer, sodium, and fluid retention, hypertension, hyperglycemia, impaired wound healing endocrine abnormality increased susceptibility to infection	• Not to be stopped abruptly • Watch for signs of infection and • Fluid retention
Promethazine (Phenargan)	Oral– IM, IV, rectal, 25 mg 6 hourly, 25 mg to 5th hourly, IM or IV	Vertigo extrapyramidal symptoms	Antiemetic	Sedation, drowsiness, etc.	Look for any drowsiness, if IV vein look for any rashes, even gangrene

Contd...

Contd...

Name/trade name	*Dosage/route*	*Indication*	*Action*	*Side effects*	*Nursing responsibility*
Propranolol (Inderal)	40-240 mg in divided doses	Tremors, migraine ataxia	Nonspecific beta adrenergic blocker	Hypotension, bradycardia, bronchospasm, hypoglycemia, impotence	Not to be used to asthmatic and diabetic patients
Pyrazinamide	15-25 mg/kg/day orally	2nd line of treatment for TB	Antituberculosis	Long-term usage can cause deafness	—
Rifampicin	600 mg/day–orally	1st line treatment for TB	Antituberculosis	Nausea, vomiting	Should advice to take continuously
Sodium valproate	500 mg/day increased to maximum 3000 mg/day adults 10-40 mg/kg/day for children	Typical absence Myoclonic seizure Febrile seizure	Possibility of increased GABA concentration	Anorexia, nausea, dizziness, confusion, weight gain, alopacia, thrombocytopenia	Look for side effects
Streptomycin	15 mg/kg/day – IM	2nd line of treatment for TB	Antituberculosis	Long-term usage can cause deafness	—
Symmetrel (Amantadine)	100-300 mg PO twice a day	Parkinson's disease	Increases the dopamine release, blocks dopamine reuptake and stimulates dopamine receptors	Ankle edema, confusion, hallucination, insomnia	—

Contd...

Contd...

Name/trade name	*Dosage/route*	*Indication*	*Action*	*Side effects*	*Nursing responsibility*
Tegretol (Carbamazepine)	300-1200 mg daily in divided dose 3-4 times a day Starting dose may be 200 mg tds	Partial and generalized seizures, trigeminal neuralgia	Reduces polysynaptic responses and blocks post-titanic potentiation	Double or blurred vision dizziness, GI upsets, agranulocytosis, ataxia	• Frequent drug level evaluation to be carried out • Observe for side effects like visual disturbances, GI problems
Tensilon (Edrophonium)	2 mg IV test dose 8 mg IV after 45 seconds	Evaluation for myasthenia gravis	Short acting anticholinesterase	Nausea, bradycardia erythemia	• Drug to be used only when all the emergency drugs and equipments are kept ready
Trihexyphenidyl HCl (Pacetone, Artane)	1-5 mg bd or tid	Parkinson disease, idiopathic torsion dystonia	Anticholinergic	Visual blurring, dry mouth, urinary retention	Dosage is decreased in pregnancy
Warfarin (Coumadine)	To begin with 4 mg orally/day Later dose adjusted accordingly	Stroke prophylaxis	Inhibits vitamin K, dependent clotting factor	Bleeding, rash, skin necrosis	• Regular evaluation of PT • Watch for any bleeding and symptoms of internal bleeding
Zidovudine	100 mg 4th hourly or 200 mg 8th hourly –oral	Asymptomatic and symptomatic patients with HIV	Inhibits HIV replication	—	-do-

24

Rehabilitation of Patients with Neurological and Neurosurgical Problems—Nurses' Role

Rehabilitation is a dynamic process through which a person is assisted to achieve optimal physical, emotional, psychological, social and vocational potential and to maintain dignity, self-respect and quality of life that is as self-fulfilling and satisfying as possible.

Rehabilitation refers to a continuum of functional restoration. Rehabilitation is considered as the one of the functions of holistic approach of the health team to bring a sick person to his original condition as far and as early as possible. In some instances complete recovery and functional restoration is possible, e.g. mild cerebral concussion. But in other instances like multiple sclerosis no complete functional restoration is possible but the rehabilitation program can optimize the quality of life through health promotion, symptom management, prevention of complications and patient and relative education to promote independence for longest possible lifetime. As the disease progresses, rehabilitation offers alternate ways of carrying out activities of daily living (ADL) with adaptive devices and alternate methods of performing skilled acts.

Nurse as a Team Member

Nurse is one of the team members of rehabilitation. Other members of the team are:

- Doctors
- Physiotherapist
- Occupational therapist
- Sociologists
- Psychologists

- Religious organization
- Dietician
- Speech therapist
- Anesthetist.

Functions of Rehabilitation Nurses

These can be listed as

1. Assessment
2. Nursing diagnoses
3. Nursing intervention
4. Planning for discharge
5. Care in the community—by community nursing.

Assessment

Generally the patients who need rehabilitation can be categorized into three groups as:

- Patients with impairment
- Patients with disability
- Patients with handicap.

Definitions

Impairment: Loss or abnormality of psychological, physiological or anatomical structure or function at organ level—the symptoms and signs.

Disability: The restriction or lack of ability to perform an activity in a normal manner—the functional consequences.

Handicap: The disadvantage, due to impairment or disability, that limits or prevents fulfillment of a 'normal' role—the social and societal consequences.

Assessment by nurse can be with following dimensions:

1. Biological
2. Cognitive
3. Social
4. Psychological
5. Family
6. Communication.

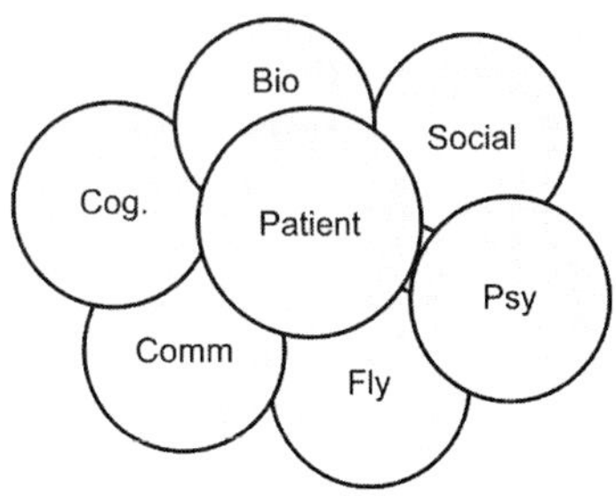

Sources of Data

1. The client

2. Friends and family
3. Medical records
4. Diagnostic tests
5. Functional and physical test batteries and assessment scales.
   Assessment may be done using various scales available.

Assessment of Family

Knowledge about patient condition

- Cooperation
- Family living patterns
- Financial ability
- Application of principles of general hygiene.
- Assessment of age related problems. Some assessment should be done to each patient as each age group can have specific problems.
- Assessment related to disease which claims his rehabilitation according to the prognosis of the disease.

There are several assessment methods that are used for specific disease like stroke, multiple scleroses, Parkinson's disease, head injury and spinal injury to test the severity of or effects of illness.

Nursing Diagnoses

Common nursing diagnoses are:

- Airway ineffective
- Cardiac output decreased
- Communication impaired
- Fluid volume deficit
- Hypothermia
- Hyperthermia
- Incontinence
- Risk for infection
- Nutrition altered
- Skin integrity impaired
- Risk for trauma
- Sleep pattern disturbance
- Deficits in ADL
- Impaired swallowing
- Impaired memory
- Impaired mobility
- Altered thought process.

Nursing Intervention

They vary quite a lot depending upon the condition of the patient, available resources and policies of the individual institutions.

Planning for Discharge

The hospitals, where there is a well-equipped rehabilitation center, patient can be kept for considerably long duration. If not, patient is discharged from the ward with lot of deficits or functional problems. So the nurse is the person who can train the patient and relatives to the maximum, how to manage the patient and use the available resources at home. This training should be individually tailored as intensity of the problem in each individual is different, the understanding of the relatives and the resources available for them are different.

Community Care

If the nurse is available in the community, she has to visit the home to see the facilities available. Assess and assist them to alter the environment to facilitate the patient to have maximum speedy recovery.

Frequent visits are necessary in the beginning and can be reduced as the patient improves and become independent. Government and Nongovernment organizations can be approached for further management.

Some general principles in rehabilitating nursing:

1. Rehabilitation should start from the day patient comes to hospital.
2. Each individual is different and their needs are different.
3. Planning should be individually tailored.
4. Individual has the right for privacy, deserves dignity.
5. Planning should be built on individual patient's personalities and needs.
6. Team-work is always necessary to make the rehabilitation effective.
7. Recreation, leisure and social interaction are to be included in the rehabilitation.

To have health problems are common or unavoidable. Some disease conditions are totally curable and individuals come back to normal. But other conditions leave the individuals with some deficits physically, psychologically, socially or financially. So the rehabilitation has very important and pivotal role to bring the diseased individuals back to normal as much and as early as possible. So the functions of a nurse in rehabilitation is as important as in any other role in the health care.

25

Prevention of Neurological and Neurosurgical Conditions—Nurses' Role

There are a few neurological and neurosurgical conditions which can be prevented completely. Some others can be identified in time and prevent further complications in other systems of the body. Still others are there, where careful action, continuous treatment and rigid follow-up can prevent recurrence. Some conditions can have their effect on the family members, their financial, social and professional life. As a member of the health team, the nurse has a duty in preventing such conditions at every stage. For convenient discussion, the neurological and neurosurgical conditions which can be prevented completely or partially are grouped as follows:

Neurosurgical Conditions

1. Congenital abnormalities/developmental disorders
2. Head injuries
3. Spinal injuries.

Neurological Conditions

1. Epilepsy/convulsions
2. Stroke and CVT
3. Infections of the nervous system
4. Dementia and degenerative diseases
5. Peripheral neuropathy.

In the following pages, the measures that a nurse can take to prevent the neurological condition are given briefly.

Congenital Abnormalities/Developmental Disorders

- Discourage consanguineous marriages which can trigger the incidental rate of congenital abnormalities.

- Avoid infection during pregnancy especially in 1st trimester.
- Avoid drugs like antibiotics, hormones during the 1st trimester of pregnancy.
- Exposure to X-rays, scan can be avoided during pregnancy.
- Any fall, injuries, even blunt injuries to abdomen during pregnancy should be avoided and if happened to be reported to the concerned doctor.
- Drug abuse also should be avoided.
- Once labor starts, special attention to be taken to prevent prolonged labor, difficult labor, fetus distress, instrumental deliveries, etc.
- Soon after the child is born, a pediatrician is expected to examine the child to detect any abnormalities and treat quickly to prevent further complications.

Head Injuries

Though the nurses have little direct role in preventing head injuries, community nurse has much to do in this area. Different medias can be used to make the people aware about the problems related to head injuries and measures to prevent them. They can be:

- Use helmet while riding two wheelers.
- Do not overload the vehicle to prevent imbalance and cause accidents.
- Do not ride or drive vehicles under the influence of alcohol or sedative drugs.
- Always keep first aid articles to prevent further complications in case of occurrence of accidents.
- Individuals should have identity cards to inform the relatives as early as possible.
- Identity card can have the informations like blood group, drugs which they are allergic to if any, and any drugs they are on.
- Never get into speedy vehicles.
- Never get into overloaded public transports.
- Take opportunities to make the children aware about the safety measures while they play, ride and even walk on the road.
- Slippery floors of rooms or toilets can cause fall of elderly people. So enough precaution should be taken when there are elderly people at home.

Spinal Injuries

Spinal injuries can be caused alone or along with head injury, so the criteria for the prevention of occurrence can be same as in case of head injury. But prevention of further complication of spinal injury is more important. They are:

At the site of the incident

- Use firm board or frame to support the spine.
- Immobilize the patient as far as possible.
- Base or the frame along with patient is shifted to and from wherever the patient is to be transported, not the patient alone. In other words patient is not lifted from the base or frame.

At the hospital

- Use collar, pelvic frame and so on if necessary.
- Complete bedrest is given until complete healing occurs.
- Each system of the body to be taken care as complication can occur on any part of the body according to the spinal region involved during injury.
- The complications expected and prevented are:
    - i. Respiratory infection
    - ii. Pressure sores
    - iii. Contractures
    - iv. Footdrop
    - v. Bladder dysfunction leading to upper urinary tract failure
    - vi. Bowel dysfunction which also can trigger the urinary tract problems and pressure sores
    - vii. Malnutrition if the chewing and swallowing actions are defective.

On discharge

- Patient and family should be given enough social, financial rehabilitative support, if the patient has to live with deficits which are chronic or permanent in nature.

Convulsion and Epilepsy

Public teaching can be according to the known causes of epilepsy/ convulsion.

During antenatal period

- Prevent infection.
- Avoid injuries.

- Have balanced diet with increase in calcium.
- Avoid any drug abuse.

Intranatal

- Avoid prolonged and difficult deliveries to prevent decreased O_2 supply to the fetus.
- Any injury during instrumental delivery may be avoided.

Postnatal

- Suctioning of throat of the child is necessary to prevent hypoxia to brain.
- Immediate postnatal injuries to be avoided.
- Any infection to be taken care of immediately.
- Warm water bath is recommended than hot water bath.

When the child has increased body temperature

- Parents should be advised that never the body temperature should go beyond 102° F. They can use measures like tepid sponge, putting fan on, keep the child under running tap, give paracetamol to control the fever and consult the physician.
- Never cover the child with bed sheets or blanket. Once it is diagnosed as febrile convulsions or epilepsy, treatment should be for a long time. So parents should be instructed to complete the course of medication and do the follow-up rigidly.
- Infections like TB, meningitis, cisticercosis, granulomas, head injuries or increased intracranial pressure are causes of convulsion. Public can be made aware of the prognosis and course of treatment and complications when treatment is inadequate in the above said conditions.

Stroke and CVT

Health talk, individually or through media can help the people to prevent stroke and CVT partially. The measures are:

- To have regular medical check-up especially above 40 years of age. Because people above 40 years of age are prone to get systemic diseases like increased blood pressure, increased blood sugar and other systemic diseases which can directly or indirectly cause stroke.
- Avoid too much fatty/oily food.
- Encourage enough physical activities.
- Discourage smoking especially heavy smoking.
- Oral contraceptives can be avoided or to be taken with physician's instruction only.

- Once increased blood pressure, increased blood sugar or any systemic diseases is diagnosed, the treatment should be continued and follow-up is absolute necessary.
- Stress to be avoided and treated early.
- Stress management can be taught to the individuals and to the public.

CVT can be prevented partially by

- Good antenatal care.
- Hospital delivery.
- Plenty of intake of fluids to the mother in the postnatal period.
- Early ambulation after delivery.
- Tight bandages around the abdomen to be avoided during postnatal period.
- Any infection to the mother during postnatal period to be avoided and treated effectively if it occurs to avoid CVT.

Infections of Nervous System

Infections to nervous system can be with virus, bacteria, parasites or HIV viruses. Different measures can be taken in order to prevent them, and most of them can be prevented completely.

Health awareness camps can be conducted or media like TV, newspaper can be used to propagate the safety measures.

- Repeated common cold needs careful medical attention.
- Any infection to oral cavity to be treated as early as possible as it can lead to ear infection.
- Any ear infection to be attended immediately as it can lead to middle ear infection, meningitis, encephalitis, etc.
- Advice not to take bath in infected ponds, pools, etc.
- Avoid using sharp pens, pencils, etc. to clean the ear which can cause rupture of tympanic membrane and further infection to brain and its coverings.
- Tuberculosis of any organ to be treated till the course of medication is completed, as it can cause meningitis, myelitis, increased ICP, convulsions, etc.
- Public can be given the awareness of not to use the uncooked meat especially pork as it can cause cisticercosis.
- Vegetables and fruits should be washed properly especially when they are eaten uncooked, as it can infect the individuals with *Taenia solium*.

- People can be educated to prevent HIV infection. The guidelines may be:
  i. Do not have sex with unknown people, if so use condom.
  ii. Do not have multiple sex partners.
  iii. Select recognized registered hospitals or clinics to have blood transfusions, intramuscular injections or intravenous injections where only disposable sets are used.
  iv. Be careful to select the hospitals while donating blood (to use only sterile equipments).
  v. Avoid contact with any body fluids, like vaginal secretions, semen serum from wounds, cerebrospinal fluid of any person without proper protection.
  vi. Avoid contact with blood of any individuals without proper protections.
  vii. It is advisable to go for investigations to confirm that future spouses are not infected with HIV.

Dementia

Dementia is an outcome of normal aging. But there are some conditions which can cause early aging which can be prevented partially. The precautions can be:

- Regular medical check-up to see the irregularities in blood pressure, diabetes, serum cholesterol and imbalances in renal and liver function. Once if any conditions are identified, proper medication to be continued and do the follow-up regularly.
- As sexually transmitted diseases like syphilis, gonorrhea and AIDS can make degeneration faster, investigations should be done and to be treated.
- Make the people aware of the consequences of alcoholisms which can cause early degeneration of brain and cause dementia. So that they may be motivated to stop or decrease the alcohol consumption.
- Educate the public the importance of balanced diet to avoid early degenerative changes in the brain.
- Public can be made aware of expected problems in each stages of life and guidelines to solve the problems themselves or to approach professional individuals or organizations.
- Positive coping mechanism and stress reduction techniques to be taught to the common people individually or through mass media.

- People with degenerative disorders can be given knowledge for early identification of relapsing symptoms and get medical treatment.
- Educate the people to live effectively and efficiently as far as possible even with permanent deficits.

Peripheral Neuropathy

Detection and treatment of all systemic diseases like diabetes, increased blood pressure, abnormal renal or liver functions, vitamin deficits, endocrine disorders are to be recommended.

- As alcoholism is the main cause of peripheral neuropathy in elderly people, special campaign can be arranged to give the public, the awareness to abstain from alcohol.
- Coloured toys made of lead paint to be avoided as the lead can cause peripheral neuropathy.
- Any type of tinkling, numbness, burning, prickling sensation and peripheral to be reported.

The nurses' role in preventing neurological and neurosurgical conditions can be summarized in the following lines.

1. Prevent certain conditions from occurring in the nervous system.
2. Prevent the complications of these conditions to other systems by early identification and effective treatment.
3. Prevent the recurrence by effective treatment and rigid follow-up.
4. Prevent the consequences of these conditions to the financial, social, professional life of the individual and their family.

26

Summary of Common Problems, Nursing Diagnosis and Interventions in Neuroscience Nursing

Table 26.1: Common problems in neuroscience nursing

Sl.No.	*Problems identified*	*Nursing diagnosis*	*Nursing intervention*
1.	Unable to breath	Ineffective airway clearance related to unconsciousness or ineffective cough reflex	• Turn the patient to one side • Elevate the head end of the bed to 30° • Suction as necessary • Provide chest physiotherapy • Encourage coughing and deep breathing exercise if patient is conscious • Give humidified oxygen therapy
2.	Unstable vital signs	Altered tissue perfusion, cerebral/respiratory tract ischemia, cerebral edema or increased ICP	Monitor vital and neurological signs Elevate the head end of the bed to 30° angle Maintain normothermia Avoid activities which increases ICP, e.g. coughing constipation
3.	Unable to communicate	Impaired verbal communication	Assess the type of communication deficit present Develop appropriate method for communication
4.	Physical weakness	Inadequate nutrition related to decreased intake	1. Determine reasons for inadequate intake and treat them 2. Provide food of patient's choice

Contd....

Sl.No.	Problems identified	Nursing diagnosis	Nursing intervention
			3. Provide nutrition and suppliment light small frequent meal 4. Assess the need for tube feeding or parenteral nutrition
5.	Not able to do ADL	Self-care deficit related to cognitive and motor impairment	• Assess the ability to complete ADL • Provide assistance to perform ADL if necessary
6.	Unable to walk steadily	Risk for injury related to impaired cognitive and motor function	• Instruct the patient not to move around without assistance • Give supportive appliances like walking stick, walker etc. Keep constant watch on the patient
7.	Not interacting with others	Impaired social interaction due to impaired physical mobility or cognitive deficits	• Assess the patient's mental and physical abilities • Help them to move around with help of supportive measures • Determine the types of activities possible to the current level of functioning and assist them to perform it. • Assist patient and family to plan the activities to stimulate interaction • Encourage visitors • Arrange group interaction sessions in the ward
8.	Unstable mood	Altered coping mechanism	• Assess current coping of patients and family • Assist patient in identifying specific stressors and resolutions to the problems • Refer to appropriate health agencies
9.	Incontinence of urine	Altered bladder function	• Monitor frequency and amount of urine voided • Identify the type of bladder problem present

Contd....

Sl.No.	*Problems identified*	*Nursing diagnosis*	*Nursing intervention*
			• Provide continuous urinary drainage • Institute appropriate program for the individual patients
10.	Inability to perform normal sexual activity	Sexual dysfunction	• Assess the presence of dysfunction • Assist them to realize the problem and help them to accept it • Make referral if necessary for the patient and sexual partner
11.	Anxiety prior to surgery	Knowledge deficit related to up coming surgery	• Explain the need for surgery and procedure at the level of patient understanding • Explain the prognosis after the surgery and role of the patient before and after surgery
12.	Worried about the surgery	Fear related to upcoming surgery	• Allow the patient to express the feelings • Correct if any miscon-ceptions • Provide emotional and psychological support • Help the patient to identify fears and discuss them • Reassure the patient
13.	Dehydration	Risk for fluid volume deficit	• Maintain intake/output record • Report a urinary output of 200 ml/hour or more for 2 consecutive hour • Encourage fluid intake if the patient is able to consume orally, if not administer IV fluids
14.	Dry mouth	Altered oral mucous membrane related to mouth breathing	• Offer mouth care frequently
15.	Long-term hospitalization	Risk for infection	• Good handwashing • Follow aseptic techniques while doing any procedure • Food prepared to be served under sanitary condition

Contd..

Sl.No.	Problems identified	Nursing diagnosis	Nursing intervention
			• Symptoms of fever chills local signs of infection are promptly evaluated and treated • Catheter sites and IV sites to be taken care properly • Appropriate personal hygiene to be given
16.	Bedridden for long time	Impaired skin integrity/tissue integrity	• Change of position every 2 hours. Providing proper care to bony prominences of the body • Prevent incontinence of urine and motion • Keep the patient dry all the time • Provide nutritious food • Provide range of motion exercises • Use special mattress if needed
17.	Immobility	Risk of contractures and footdrop and chances of disuse syndrome	• Provide active and passive exercises • Ambulate as early as possible • Provide chest physiotherapy and suction if necessary • Encourage deep breathing exercises
18.	Not able to move	Impaired physical mobility	• Assess the type and degree of impairment • Provide slings, braces support shoes and so on as necessary • Teach the patient alternate methods of mobility • Provide for range of motion exercises 4 times a day
19.	Fever	Hyperthermia related to infection inflammation and pressure on the hypothalamus	• Remove excess bed clothes • Apply cool wet cloth to the head • Provide tepid water bath as necessary • Assess the need for use of antipyretic drugs and administer

Contd..

Sl.No.	*Problems identified*	*Nursing diagnosis*	*Nursing intervention*
20.	Pain	Pain (Headache, neck, back pain)	• Assess the type, location and specific characteristics of headache • Apply ice cap or cold or wet cloth to the patient head for comfort • Darken the patient room • Administer analgesic as ordered
21.	Restlessness	Sensory/perceptual alteration due to meningeal irritation	• Note any evidence of discomfort due to direct light • Maintain a darkened room
22.	C/o headache and confused	High-risk for injury seizure activity secondary to cerebral irritation	• Maintain seizure precautions • Monitor patient for any signs of seizure activities and document in the chart • Administer anticonvulsant • Provide side rail cot
23.	Sleeplessness	Sleep pattern disturbance	• Document the sleep wakefulness pattern • Identify the factors that prevent adequate sleep • Identify and correct the misconceptions • Avoid sleeping during day • Provide sedation if necessary only in the late night • Decrease environmental stimuli at night • Make the patient comfortable
24.	Low self-esteem	Self-concept disturbance/ personal identity disturbance	• Gain the confidence of patient through good interpersonal relationship (IPR) • Allow expression of feelings • Be supportive and assist in developing strategies to deal with the problem • Identify support groups in the hospital and community • Make appropriate referrals
25.	Misconceptions regarding the illness	Knowledge deficit	• Assess the patient knowledge about the illness

Contd..

Sl.No.	Problems identified	Nursing diagnosis	Nursing intervention
			• Provide necessary information about illness to the patient and family • Provide necessary information about available resources
26.	Unable to cough	Risk for aspiration	• Turn the patient to one side • Introduce airway • Nothing per mouth is given • Suction the throat as necessary
27.	Pain in the leg while resting	Risk of deep vein thrombosis	• Provide crape bandage or stockings • Administer heparin if not contraindicated • Elevate the leg to 30° angle
28.	Distention of urinary bladder	Urinary retention	• Apply hot and cold compress on the abdomen • Open the tap and encourage the patient to pass urine • Catheterize if necessary

Other Commonly Used Nursing Diagnosis are

- Physical mobility impaired
- Thought processes altered
- Sensory perception altered
- Individual coping impaired
- Adjustment impaired
- Diversional activity deficits
- Risk of disuse syndrome
- Risk of skin integrity impaired
- Risk for aspiration
- Impaired gas exchange
- Fluid volume deficits
- Social isolation
- Body image disturbance.

Nursing interventions in neurological and neurosurgical nursing is mainly aimed

1. To avoid increased ICP
2. To avoid deterioration of conscious level
3. To limit the neurological deficits.

These objectives should be combined with the nursing interventions in general hospitals.

27

Nursing Management of Patients with Ventilator

Neurology is a specialized branch of medicine which deals with conditions affecting the nervous system. But many patients admitted in Neurocenter need ventilator care which directly supports the respiratory system. Because the interdependency of nervous system and respiratory system is very high and complex, so the nurses working in Neurocenter need to know the normal physiology of both these systems with the expected conditions where the ventilator care is indicated. They are also to be equipped with the knowledge and skill to manage these machines which play an important place in the management and progress of these patients.

CONDITIONS NEED VENTILATOR CARE AND MANAGEMENT

Nursing care is quite challenging because unattended respiratory problems can cause neurological deterioration but at the same time therapeutic procedures aimed at optimizing the respiratory function, can have some adverse effects on the neurological pathway. A thorough understanding of the intricate balance is the key to successful management of these patients.

Before going to the management, let we know how does the normal respiration occur.

Flow chart 27.1: Pathway of normal respiration

Medullary center—Pons

↓

Spinal cord

↓

Diaphragm

↓

Contd..

Respiratory muscles
↓
Myoneural junction
↓
Thoracic case/cage ↑ size
↓
Air entry → to thoracic cage
↓
Alveoli
↓
Exchange of gases

From the above Flow chart it can be concluded that the causes of respiratory problems can be from Medullary-CNS disorders like:

- Head Injury
- Poisoning
  Trauma of any other cause.
- Spinal Cord – Injury
  – Tumors
- Peripheral nerves – GB syndrome
- Neuromuscular function – Myasthenia gravis
  – Botulism (food poisoning)
- Respiratory muscle – Myopathies
- Thoracic cage – Kyphoscoliosis
  – Airway obstruction
- Lung – Alveoli collapse injury.

Diagnosis of respiratory failures is done by:

1. Signs of respiratory distress
   - All distress will have failure but all failure may not have distress.
   - Distress can be watched by – flaring of nostrils
   - Inverted costal muscles
2. Signs of hypoxia like:
   - Restlessness
   - Sweating
   - ↑ BP leading to ↓ BP
   - Tachycardia
   - Cyanosis

3. Investigations
   - X-ray chest
   - Arterial blood gas analysis
   - Normal PCO_2 – 100 mm of Hg
     - PCO_2 – 70 mm of Hg for elder
     - $PaCO_2$ – 40 mm of Hg

Treatment

For hypoxia – O_2 given by
- Nasal catheter
- Master
- Tents

For ventilator failure – C $\downarrow$ PCO_2 and $\uparrow$ $PaCO_2$
– Give O_2 by ventilator

Indication for ventilator connection.
1. $PaCO_2 < 60$ mm of Hg in spite of CO_2 therapy
2. $PaCO_2 > 45$ mm of Hg
3. Vital capacity is < 1 liter or 15 ml/kg.

Connection to ventilator can be:
1. By oral endotracheal tube
2. By nasal endotracheal tube
3. Tracheotomy.

Size of the tube is decided by the age and sex of the patient. The normal calculation is:
- Male adult—size 8 to 10
- Female—size 7 to 8.5
- Children up to 6 years $= \frac{\text{Age}}{3} + 3.5$
- Children from 6 – 12 years $= \frac{\text{Age}}{4} + 4.5$

Advantages and Disadvantages of Oral and Nasal Endotracheal Tubes

Oral	*Nasal*
• Easy to intubate	• Difficult to intubate
• Uncomfortable for the patient	• Comparatively comfortable
• Oral hygiene is difficult	• Easy oral hygiene
• Infection is low	• Infection is high

Types of Ventilators

1. Negative pressure ventilators
2. Positive pressure ventilators
    - Volume cycled
    - Pressure cycled
    - Flow cycled
    - Time cycled.

Modes of Mechanical Ventilator

Mode refers to how the ventilator helps to patient to relate his/her own effort to ventilate. Different modes are available in different machines. Corresponding to the ability of the patient's own effort. They are:

- Controlled mandatory ventilator
- Assist control mandatory ventilator
- Synchronized intermittent mandatory ventilator
- Pressure support ventilator
- Pressure controlled ventilator
- Biphasic positive air pressure ventilator.

Complications of Mechanical Ventilator

1. Decreased cardiac output
2. Barotrauma
3. Nosocomial infection.

Management

- Prevent cross infection
- Prevent risk for aspiration
- Limit suctioning
- Observe sterile techniques while doing suctioning
- Avoid pooling of condensation in the tubing
- Avoid condensed water entering to humidifier and to the ETT
- Fluid intake to be balanced, nutrition to be taken care of
- Passive/Active exercises to avoid complications.

Common Nursing Problems Identified in Neuro ICU

1. Impaired spontaneous ventilation
2. Impaired gas exchange
3. Ineffective breathing pattern

4. Risk for infection
5. Fear and anxiety
6. Impaired verbal communication
7. Impaired sleep-wake cycle
8. Impaired balance nutrition.

Nursing Management

- Check the ventilator frequently to see the placement of E.T.T, setting of ventilator alarm and connections.
- Watch for any sign of distress and fighting with the ventilator.
- Ensure adequate humidification.
- For any airway obstruction use AMBU bag to inflate lung with 100 percent oxygen for short time and suction to clear the airway.

Chest physio, postural drainage changing the position of patient is advised

- Monitor ABG
- Hyperventilate the patient before and after suctioning.
- Other general nursing principles can be used to reduce infection, fear and anxiety, to maintain nutritional, prevent bedsore, and problems of.........nation, etc.

Weaning from Ventilator

Weaning is generally started when the original pathology is corrected and pulmonary function is improved. Weaning is done gradually and pulling the patient intermittently from ventilator, looking at the patient's condition each time of partial weaning. Outcome of NICU patients depends upon the angenal pathology of disease. If primary pathology is reversible the outcome is good. For example, GB syndrome, myasthenia gravis, there are irreversible conditions like permanent damage to respiratory center, respiratory organs or respiratory muscles. The progress and good outcome of these conditions depend mainly on the nursing management.

Bibliography

1. A handbook for caregivers of those suffering from dementia (1999). A souvenir released on the occasion of Southzone Conference of Alzheimer's and Related Disorders Society of India.
2. Alexander MF, Fanceh JN. In: Rungman PJ (Ed). 'Nursing practice' hospital and home (2nd edn). Churchill Livingstone; 2000.
3. Alexander MF, Josephine F, Runciman. 'Nursing practice' (2nd edn). Churchill Livingstone; 2000.
4. Arunodaya, G. Emergencies in epilepsy. In: Manual on Epilepsy for Medical Practitioner NIMHANS, Bangalore; 1999.
5. Bickerstaff, Edwin R, Peter H, Seh RR. Neurology (3rd edn). London. Hodder and Stoughton.
6. Bousser G, Barnett JM. Cerebral venous thrombosis, stroke: pathophysiology, diagnosis and management, 4th edn.
7. Campbell C. Acoustic neuroma nursing implications related to surgical management. Journal of Neuroscience Nursing; 1991: 23(1).
8. Chopra JS. Neurology in tropics. BI Churchill Livingstone; 1999.
9. Conway BL. Neurological and neurosurgical nursing Rutkawski (8th edn). CV Mosby; 1982.
10. Coralease, Ethel. Diagnosing urinary incontinence. Neuroscience Nursing; 1989: 14(6).
11. Current management of incontinence. Indian Continence Foundation; 1999.
12. Dasgupta PC, Godwen HR, Flower CJ. The 'queen square bladder stimulation': A device for assisting emptying of neurogenic bladder. British Journal of Urology; 1997.
13. Davis S, Connor S'O'. Rehabilitation nursing foundations for practice. Baillier's Tindall, Edinburgh, London; 1999.
14. Doris Smith Suddarth. The Lippincott manual of nursing practice (5th edn). Philadelphia, JB Lippincott Company; 1992.
15. Doughlous A. Nursing and neuroscience (1st edn). Longman: Suigpore Pub Pvt Ltd; 1988.
16. Drug today. (1999) July-Sep.
17. Dylantt S, Peter H. "Tackling incontinence". Nursing Times, 1990; 86(10).

18. Eisenberg L. Preventing mental neurological and psychosocial disorders. World Health Forum 8; 1987.
19. Evelyn P. Anatomy and physiology for nurses (15th edn). Calcutta Oxford University Press; 1977.
20. Gami NK. Bedside approach to clinical neurology (2nd edn). Jaypee Publication; 1998.
21. Global programme on AIDS, HIV prevention and care, teaching modules for nurses and midwives. World Health Organisation.
22. Gourie Devi M, Gururaj G, Satishchandra P. Neuroepidemiology in India. A perspective in recent advances in tropical neurology. Rose FC (Ed.). Elsevier Science, 1995. pp. 17-30.
23. Hicky J. Clinical practice of neurological and neurosurgical nursing (2nd and 4th edn). JB Lippincott.
24. Isaac MK, Chandrasekhar CR, Srinivasamurthy R. Manual of mental health for medical officers. National Institute of Mental Health and Neurosciences. Bangalore; 1985-87.
25. Joan Luck Mann MA, Swceny K. Saunder's manual of nursing care. WB Saunders Company; 1997.
26. Joanne HV. The clinical practice of neurological and neurosurgical nursing (2nd and 4th edn). Philadelphia, Lippincott; 1977.
27. Johnson. "From Incontinence to confidence". American Journal of Nursing; 2000. 2: p. 100.
28. Kilmber, Pole's GS. Anatomy and physiology (16th edn). New Delhi, Amarind Publishers; 1978.
29. Lous, Collar, Sharon Martek Louis and Idolia Cox Coller. Medical surgical nursing. Mosby's year book; 1992.
30. Manley K, Bellman L. Surgical nursing advance practice. Churchill Livingstone; 2000.
31. Marshall, Mayer. On call neurology. WB Saunders Company, 1998.
32. Martin A Samuels. Manual of neurology. Little Brown and Company: Boston; 1991.
33. Mitchell, Hodges, Muwaswes, Wallak. AANN's neuroscience nursing phenomena and practice. Appleton and Lange. California; 1988 and 1992.
34. Mosby's Medical Dictionary. Galgotia Publications; 1988: 367-388.
35. Owens, Carini. A textbook of neurological and neurosurgical nursing (17th edn). Published by the CV Mosby Company.
36. Peattie PI, Walker S. Understanding of nursing care (4th edn). ELBS; 1995.
37. Price WB, Hetty DeV. A quick and easy guide to neurological assessment. Journal of Neurosurgical Nursing. 1985; 5:17.
38. Samuels A. Manual of neurologic therapeutics (5th edn). Little Brown and Company. Boston, New York; 1995.

39. Satishchandra P, Gourie Devi M. Manual on epilepsy for medical officers. NIMHANS, Bangalore; 1999 (Epilepsy Control Programme Sponsored by WHO).

40. Satishchandra P. Clinical characteristics of epilepsy in manual on epilepsy for medical officer. In: Satishchandra P, Gourie Devi M (Eds): NIMHANS, Bangalore; 1999.

41. Scherer JC, RNMS: Lippincott's nurse's drug manual. Philadelphia, JB Lippincott Company; 1985.

42. Sotelo J, DelBrutto OH. Neurocysticercosis in neurology in tropics. Chopro JS (Ed): BI Churchill Livingstone, 1999; 229-39.

43. Srinivasan K. Cerebral venous thrombosis in neurology in tropics. Chopra JS. BI Churchill Livingstone Pvt, 1999.

44. Srinivasan R. Drug treatment epilepsy in manual on epilepsy for medical officer. Bangalore NIMHANS; 1999.

45. Therapeutic Index and Hoechst India Limited.

46. Thomas, et al. Prevalence of urinary incontinence. British Medical Journal; 1980.

47. Tomblin JB, Morris HL, Sprieslersbach DC. Diagnosis in speech—Language pathology. California, Singular Pub Group Inc.

48. Watson R. Essential science for nursing students. Bailliere Tindall with Ren: London; 1999.

49. Witherington Stress R. Urinary incontinence. A practical protocol for geriatrics; 1982.

Index

C

D

E

H

I

K

L

M

N

O

P

R

S

T

U

V

W

X